The *Natural* Estrogen Diet & Recipe Book

Ordering

Trade bookstores in the U.S. and Canada please contact:
  Publishers Group West
  1700 Fourth Street, Berkeley CA 94710
  Phone: (800) 788-3123   Fax: (800) 351-5073

For bulk orders please contact:
  Special Sales
  Hunter House Inc., PO Box 2914, Alameda CA 94501-0914
  Phone: (510) 899-5041   Fax: (510) 865-4295
  E-mail: sales@hunterhouse.com

Individuals can order our books by calling **(800) 266-5592**
or from our website at **www.hunterhouse.com**

The *Natural* Estrogen Diet & Recipe Book

Healthy Recipes for Perimenopause and Menopause

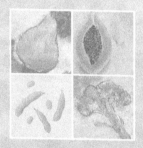

Lana Liew, M.D.

WITH LINDA OJEDA, PH.D.

Hunter House
PUBLISHERS

Library of Congress Cataloging-in-Publication Data

Liew, Lana.
  The natural estrogen diet & recipe book / Lana Liew, with Linda Ojeda.— 2nd U.S. ed.
    p. cm.
  "First published in Australia in 1998 as The natural estrogen book by Simon & Schuster."
  Includes bibliographical references and index.
  ISBN-10: 0-89793-415-6 (pbk.) — ISBN-10: 0-89793-416-4 (hc)
  ISBN-13: 978-0-89793-415-2 (pbk.)
    1. Menopause—Complications—Diet therapy—Recipes. 2. Perimenopause—Complications—Diet therapy—Recipes. 3. Menopause—Complications—Alternative treatment. 4. Menopause—Hormone therapy. 5. Menopause—Nutritional aspects. 6. Estrogen—Therapeutic use. 7. Middle aged women—Health and hygiene. I. Ojeda, Linda. II. Liew, Lana. Natural estrogen book. III. Title.
RG186.L465 2003
618.1'750654—dc21   2003012814

Project Credits

Cover Design: Brian Dittmar Graphic Design
Book Design and Production: Jinni Fontana
Recipe Editor for first edition: Naomi Wise
Recipe Editor for second edition:
    Pat Molden
Nutritional Consultant:
    Linda Yoakam, M.S., R.D., L.D.
Copy Editor: Kelley Blewster
Proofreader: Rachel E. Bernstein
Indexer: Deanna Butler

Acquisitions Editor: Jeanne Brondino
Editor: Alexandra Mummery
Publicist: Lisa E. Lee
Sales Coordinator: Jo Anne Retzlaff
Customer Service Manager:
    Christina Sverdrup
Order Fulfillment: Lakdhon Lama
Administrator: Theresa Nelson
Computer Support: Peter Eichelberger
Publisher: Kiran S. Rana

Manufactured in the United States of America

9 8 7 6 5 4 3 2   Second U.S. Edition   12 13 14 15 16

Contents

Foreword

The latest focus in nutrition research is on phytoestrogens. Phytoestrogens are a diverse group of plant-derived substances that have estrogenic activity in animals. These compounds are similar to estrogens and are characterized by their ability to elicit a specific response in estrogen-sensitive tissues. There is a great deal of interest in the potential benefits of dietary phytoestrogens in hormone-dependent processes. Animals have been known to graze selectively on plants to enhance or diminish fertility. Much of the early research on phytoestrogens was done with animals and interest was induced by the observation that sheep who grazed too much on clover became infertile. Epidemiological studies have shown that the incidence of hormone-dependent diseases is significantly lower in Asian populations whose diets are high in phytoestrogen consumption. Further studies comparing native Asian women to other cultures have suggested that the high phytoestrogen content of their diets may be responsible in part for their low rate of breast cancer and the ease with which they pass through menopause.

Phytoestrogens have both weak estrogenic and antiestrogenic activity. Estradiol, our bodies' strongest estrogen, can be released from the ovary and travel to any number of target tissues, including the breast and uterus. At the breast, the estradiol can bind to the receptor site and increase cell division; at the uterus, estradiol can cause the endometrial lining to thicken. However, not all substances have a positive effect on the target tissue. Such is the case with tamoxifen, a drug used in the treatment of breast cancer. Tamoxifen can bind to the estrogen receptors of the breast without causing any increase in cell division, thereby acting as an "estrogen blocker." At the same time, it can bind to receptors in the uterus and cause proliferation of the endometrium. Tamoxifen therefore has an antiestrogenic effect on the breast, but a proestrogenic effect on the uterus.

The most commonly studied phytoestrogens include the isoflavo-noids, lignans, and coumestans found in high amounts in soybeans, flax-seed, and alfalfa, and also in many other vegetables and fruits. Much of the original research was targeted at menopausal women. Phytoestrogens have an estrogenic effect on the vaginal epithelium similar to that seen in patients treated with hormone replacement therapy. There is evidence, too, that hot flashes are resolved. Phytoestrogens also exert a cardiovas-cular-protective effect by regulating lipid levels. Dietary soy supplemen-tation has been shown to increase bone mineral density. Phytoestrogens may also protect against some types of cancer. Finally, evidence exists that there is a lower incidence of breast, colon, and prostate cancer in Asia, where soy intake is high in comparison to Western countries, where intake is relatively low.

Certainly, more studies of women using phytoestrogens need to be done to establish both their benefits and risks. However, given the bulk of information available, the use of phytoestrogens in a well-balanced diet may be considered a relatively safe method of effecting estrogen activity.

— Dr. Randall E. Fray, M.B., Ch.B., F.R.C.O.G., F.R.A.C.O.G.
Bankstown, Australia

Preface to the Second Edition

Hormone replacement therapy (HRT) remains a hot topic since the release of the first edition of *The* Natural *Estrogen Diet* in 1999. In July 2002, HRT broke news when the investigators of the Women's Health Initiative (WHI) published their findings in *The Journal of the American Medical Association.* The randomized, controlled study on the risks and benefits of combined HRT in healthy postmenopausal women had to be terminated three years prematurely due to an observed significant increase in breast cancer, stroke, coronary heart disease, pulmonary embolism (lung clots), and DVT (clots in the deep veins of the legs) amongst the group of women (8,506) who were given oral combined HRT when compared to the placebo group (8,102 women taking blank tablets). The authors also reported the benefits of fewer colon cancers and fewer hip fractures in the treated group. The other arm of the study, comparing oral estrogen only with placebo, is still continuing, hopefully until March 2005 when we'll learn the risks and benefits of estrogen replacement therapy (ERT).

The same journal also published an article on menopausal HRT and the risk of ovarian cancer. The data for this cohort study came from records of a national breast-screening program spanning over twenty years. Although short-term combined HRT was not associated with increased risk of ovarian cancer, ERT, especially when taken for more than ten years, was associated with significant risk of the cancer. These observations need to be confirmed with a large, randomized, controlled study. Results from the second half of the WHI randomized ERT study (expected in 2005) will be important for women and their health advisors.

On 25 June 2003 authors from the WHI study released further findings regarding the effects of HRT on breast cancer and mammograms. They reported that breast cancers amongst HRT users tend to be more serious than the breast cancers in non-users. Furthermore, a higher percentage of users showed abnormalities in their mammograms.

In response to the WHI information, menopause experts and health authorities suggested that women should be aware of the risks of long-term combined HRT usage. They also advised that it is unwise to depend on HRT to prevent chronic diseases such as stroke, heart disease, and osteoporosis. It is recommended that this type of combined HRT be restricted for short-term usage in the treatment of menopausal symptoms only.

A lot of unanswered questions still exist regarding other forms of non-oral HRT. It is understandable when women who have been taking HRT for some time want to quit. After all, they know their bodies better than anyone else, and their fears of the long-term effects of HRT on their bodies are justified. It has been widely accepted that breast cancer rates increase after five years of HRT usage, be it estrogen only or combined. If a woman wants to escape the risks posed by conventional HRT, what safe options exist for her?

In the early 1990s, some very astute specialist colleagues of mine told patients to get off HRT, and warned others—who had lumpy breasts or hyperplastic endometrium or fibroids—to avoid HRT altogether. Some of these patients told me their specialist doctors were recommending that they take soy instead, suggested because of its estrogen-mimicking effects on the body.

"How does one take soy?" asked these bewildered patients. In my search for ways to help these women, my medical background and abundance of cooking experience came in handy. So did my vast firsthand experience with soy. I started to write recipes and jot down names of products they might be able to find in the supermarkets. My eldest daughter suggested that I compile the wealth of information I possessed into a book so that women other than my own patients could access the information and benefit from it.

There were few soy products in Western supermarkets until the latter half of the 1990s, when a soy explosion hit Australia. Now we have soy beverages, soy-fortified cereals, soy bread, soy macaroni, tofu, soy snacks—and the list goes on. It is so easy to eat soy these days! But soy is not the only food that can help women through their menopause. There are other foods that contain plant estrogens, which most humans can convert in the gut and absorb.

When I was training as a medical student in the early 1970s, I noted that diet was not considered to be part of the management of the disease processes and well-being of patients. I remember well the questions of patients directed to my professors about what sort of diet they should follow when they got home from the hospital. The usual reply was, "Don't worry about food. You can eat anything you like, but just take the tablets I have prescribed for you." Furthermore, when we went on our rounds to the coronary care unit (where all the heart-attack patients were monitored and treated), I could see that patients there were given bacon and eggs or sausages for breakfast. Desserts invariably comprised cheesecake, ice cream, or whipped cream on fruit salad. I am sure you will find a different situation these days when you visit coronary care wards at mealtimes. Now, every cardiologist recommends a diet low in saturated fats for cardiac patients. Dietary intervention is the primary tool in heart disease. If it fails, then drugs are prescribed, some of which will be effective and will suit the patients, but others of which will be ineffective and will impart intolerable side effects.

Such has been the change in nutrition over the past three decades. Acceptance is now widespread among medical practitioners of the impact of food and diet (as well as of exercise and other lifestyle patterns) on chronic diseases and prevention of illness. We all know that diet and food habits are hard to change. But knowledgeable and well-read individuals are open to gentle transitions as they explore new tastes and healthier foods, knowing that in the long term they are reducing their risks of developing chronic and debilitating illnesses.

The Natural *Estrogen Diet & Recipe Book: Healthy Recipes for Perimenopause and Menopause* offers a host of easy, exciting recipes to help ease your passage through the menopause years, allowing you to gain better health and freedom from the effects of hormonal irregularities that can characterize this phase of a woman's life. To reap the benefits of soy and other plant estrogens, you do not have to give up meat altogether and be a vegetarian. But, as you incorporate soy and other phytoestrogen-rich foods in your diet, you can easily reduce the proportion of animal proteins you ingest. And because the recipes in this book are so versatile, you don't have to cook separately for yourself if the rest of the family does not want to follow the estrogen diet. More than half of the recipes in this book are in fact vegetarian dishes, but you can add your favorite meat to them as well.

This new edition of *The* Natural *Estrogen Diet & Recipe Book* brings you more mouth-watering recipes, as well as an update regarding research relevant to phytoestrogens (PE) and an updated estrogen food list containing new food items (see page 18). A special feature of this edition is the inclusion of a new table in the Introduction to Part II listing the phytoestrogen content in each recipe. This will enable you to aim for the right amount of PE each day.

I am very grateful for the enormous support, constant encouragement and valuable advice from the editorial staff, especially Alexandra Mummery, Kelley Blewster, Pat Molden, Linda Yoakam, and publisher, Kiran Rana, at Hunter House, and I extend special thanks to Annie Chan and Mrs. G. Hathaway, who each contributed two of their recipes to this edition. Lastly, I thank Dr. Linda Ojeda for sharing her experience, knowledge, and research expertise in the U.S. edition.

— Lana Liew

Acknowledgments

Many scientists throughout the world have worked tirelessly in the research of phytoestrogen-containing foods and their effects on the health of men and women. They are too numerous to name, but each of them has contributed to the knowledge from which this book draws—the research into disease prevention using pure extracts of isoflavones and other plant products.

My eldest daughter, Camilla, was most enthusiastic about this book, and she spurred me on with it. Her encouragement and support are most appreciated, as is her help with research, proofreading, and tasting of the recipes.

I would also like to thank my two younger daughters, Felicia and Priscilla, who understood that their time with their mother had to be shared with a compelling project. They, too, have been most patient and supportive.

Special thanks are due to the following friends: Margaret, Bev, Nanny, Annie, Siew Fong, Stephanie, and Christopher, who have shared their recipes, thoughts, and interest. Above all, their belief and support have been vital in the development of this book. Many patients have also encouraged me along the way.

Acknowledgments of help are also due to the following: Dora Spilbergs for proofreading and useful comments; Evan Black for help with some research articles; Grahame and Lyndall Black for sustaining encouragement and interest; Jenny Chan, consultant dietitian-nutritionist (B.Sc., Masters in Nutrition and Dietetics, MDAA, APD), for her work and contribution to the analysis of the recipes in the Australian edition; Dr. Randall Fray (obstetrician and gynecologist) for his interest in and enthusiasm for the book; Professor John Eden for his helpful suggestions and comments on the original Australian draft; and David Rosenberg, Brigitta Doyle, and Siobhan O'Connor at Simon & Schuster for their assistance in the production of the Australian edition of this book.

— Lana Liew

I would like to acknowledge the many contributors who supplied recipes for our collection: the Ohio Soybean Council, the Indiana Soybean Board, VitaSoy, Azumaya, Dana Jacobi, and Laura Nilsen. A special tribute goes to Naomi Wise, for supplying a few of her own recipes and for her expert advice, and to both Naomi and Laura Harger for the Americanization of the original text. I would also like to thank the staff at Hunter House and to express particular gratitude to Wendy Low and Amy Demmon, for their painstaking efforts and patience in working with the nutritional analysis software program. And, finally, to my publisher, Kiran Rana. We did it again—another wonderful collaborative effort.

— Linda Ojeda

Important Notice

The material in this book is intended to provide information regarding nutrition and diet. Every effort has been made to provide accurate and dependable information. The contents of this book have been compiled using professional research and in consultation with medical professionals. However, health-care professionals have differing opinions, and advances in medical and scientific research are made very quickly, so some of the information may become outdated.

Therefore, the publisher, authors, and editors, and the professionals quoted in the book cannot be held responsible for any error, omission, or dated material. The authors and publisher assume no responsibility for any outcome of applying the information in this book in a program of self-care or under the care of a licensed practitioner. If you have questions concerning your nutrition or diet, or about the application of the information described in this book, consult a qualified health-care professional.

Introduction

Hormone replacement therapy (HRT) is a popular discussion topic among women, particularly those who are menopausal or perimenopausal (in the years immediately preceding the onset of menopause). HRT, which is taken in order to reduce some of the bothersome symptoms associated with menopause—hot flashes, mood swings, and the like—attempts to compensate for the falling level of estrogen production that accompanies menopause, but it is not suitable for every woman. To take HRT or not to take it? That is the driving question.

Some women are quite content with their HRT program, and they should continue with the regimen, under their doctor's supervision. However, some women have tried HRT in various combinations and forms and to their disappointment have been forced to stop because of numerous undesirable side effects. There are also those for whom HRT is definitely forbidden (women with certain kinds of cancer, for example), and thus they don't have this option. And finally, a growing number of women view menopause as a natural transition that does not require outside hormonal intervention. This book is designed to help those women who cannot tolerate hormones, cannot take hormones, or simply choose not to medicate, yet who are concerned about controlling menopausal symptoms, preserving bone integrity, and preventing heart disease. Alternatives to HRT—using natural foods and lifestyle changes—can address all of these concerns, and this book describes some of these options.

Widespread interest in nonmedical treatments for an ever-growing number of conditions is sweeping the country. Premenopausal and menopausal women who have no other option than to utilize alternative methods are clamoring for specific information and guidance. Many have read magazine articles that speak about foods that can potentially alter estrogen levels in the body, but details are scant. Which foods elicit what response, women ask, and how much of a particular food must be eaten to be effective? This book answers both these questions, based on the latest available scientific information.

The Natural *Estrogen Diet & Recipe Book* discusses a variety of foods that are rich in naturally occurring plant estrogens (known as *phytoestrogens*). It explains how these gentle estrogen-like substances can work to minimize menopausal symptoms while also benefiting the bones and the heart and possibly curbing the risk of breast cancer. Of course, nutritional information is useless unless you have a practical plan for implementing changes in your daily diet, so this book also provides a number of suggestions—from the simplest, quickest, and easiest dietary changes to more involved and creative recipes—for altering your eating habits.

The first step in the natural estrogen diet is to look at the list on page 18 of foods that contain these health-promoting substances. Consider how many of these foods are already part of your regular diet, and determine ways to integrate some of the other foods into your daily meals and snacks.

The second step is to learn about soy products. Research has found that soy contains the most potent isoflavones, a subclass of plant estrogens that are thought to be responsible for many health benefits. (For a diagram illustrating how some of the different phytoestrogens are grouped in relation to each other, see the Appendix.) For this reason, this book focuses on easy and tasty ways to add soy to your life. Soy may be foreign to your palate now, but we hope that you will remain open-minded and try something new and exciting, especially since soy has the potential for aiding your health in so many ways. Consider some of the possible benefits of soy:

- Soy has been shown to reduce hot flashes and other menopausal symptoms in some women.
- Soy has been shown to reduce coronary heart disease rates and lower high blood pressure and elevated cholesterol in human subjects.
- Soy increases bone density in postmenopausal women and may protect them from osteoporosis.

❧ Animal studies suggest that soy works as well as HRT to keep arteries to the brain free of cholesterol; thus, it may prevent stroke.

❧ Soy may help to fight breast cancer. Rates of breast cancer are lower in Asia and other regions where soy foods are eaten in large quantities.

❧ Soy may be instrumental in preventing other cancers, such as endometrial cancer in women, prostate cancer in men, and colon cancer.

What Are the Advantages of the Natural Estrogen Diet?

❧ It is completely natural, and you can use the diet without fear of contraindications or the side effects that you may experience with HRT.

❧ The foods are readily available and do not require prescriptions or a visit to a health practitioner.

❧ Phytoestrogens are present in a wide variety of healthy foods, which also contain other beneficial compounds such as natural vitamins, minerals, antioxidants, healthy fats, and fiber.

❧ Besides containing plant estrogens, some of the foods in the diet also contain plant progestins. Examples are red clover, thyme, and turmeric. Progestins are hormones that behave like progesterone. Progesterone is the other hormone produced by women in significant amounts during the second half of the menstrual cycle, and its levels also fall during perimenopause and menopause.

❧ The natural estrogen diet is less costly than HRT.

❧ The diet has psychological as well as physical benefits. You are helping yourself without taking medications or drugs in order to feel "normal."

✣ What Are the Disadvantages of ✣
the Natural Estrogen Diet?

◈ Doses are not standardized in natural or manufactured foods. Researchers are still exploring the amount of phytoestrogen that is sufficient to produce health benefits. Conventional HRT tablets and patches, on the other hand, do come in standard doses, which also require titration in many users.

◈ Changing eating habits is inconvenient for some women, who may rely on swallowing a tablet or slapping on a patch to remedy their symptoms. This could be due to an attitudinal problem or simply a lack of time.

◈ Certain foods or ingredients in the diet may be difficult to obtain or prepare.

◈ There is a general lack of knowledge about how to prepare and use the diet's foods and ingredients.

◈ Effectiveness may vary, depending upon the plant products used and also upon individual factors. Absorption of phytoestrogens, for example, depends on the amount of time food takes to pass through the intestines, the status of the gut, the presence of appropriate bacteria in the intestines, and the amount of chemicals in the plant product, which is influenced by the plant's genetic origin and the climactic and environmental conditions under which it grew.

◈ It takes a few months before individuals start to experience the benefits of the natural estrogen diet. The diet is not as fast-acting as HRT, and people often find it difficult to wait for results.

◈ Some individuals may experience flatulence (gas) during the early days of the diet if they start the diet too quickly or eat overly large portions of the foods.

◈ Contamination of plants with herbicides or modification of the genetic material of the plant product may produce previously unheard of effects.

Chapter 1, "Estrogen Foods and Menopause," discusses some of the symptoms that can accompany menopause and explains how phyto-estrogens—particularly those found in soy foods—work to alleviate menopause-related problems. Chapter 2, "Plant Hormones and Other Health Concerns for Women," discusses these substances' other promising benefits: they can help protect against heart disease, osteoporosis, and even cancer. Chapter 3 introduces you to soy foods, and Chapter 4 guides you through easy ways to integrate them into your daily diet (here, too, you'll find detailed nutritional information on soy products). Finally, Part II provides a wide range of recipes that will help you make soy and other phytoestrogen-containing foods a permanent—and delicious—part of your life.

We wish you good luck with your new dietary plan and your experimental tasting and cooking, and we also wish you many years of good health, delight, and enjoyment of the natural estrogen diet.

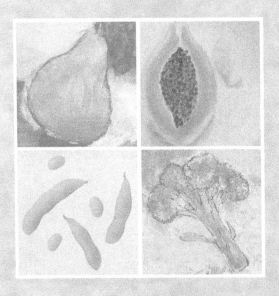

Part One

Natural
Estrogens

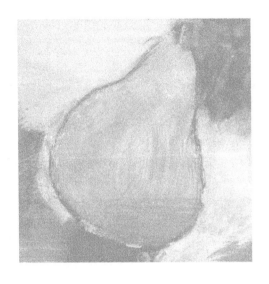

Chapter One

Estrogen Foods
& Menopause

ᗛ Symptoms of Menopause ᗛ

S ome women remember hearing about menopause from their mothers, aunts, or older friends. Others may have read about the general physical process and seen personal stories in women's magazines and newspapers or heard them on the radio or television. A smaller contingent may have even attended a full-day seminar or weekend retreat on the topic, where women shared their personal journeys and discussed facts about menopause, facts they had gone to great lengths to obtain. Whatever your source of information, you probably have a fairly good understanding of the physiology, possible symptoms, and general happenings of menopause. Still, let's just cover a few of the basics.

Menopause is the time of life when a woman's ovaries wind down and production of the hormones that have been pumping out with regularity for forty or more years slows down. For certain women, it is a smooth and relatively innocuous transition, but others find the ride somewhat bumpy, accompanied by any number of uncomfortable symptoms.

When the ovaries age or when they are removed in an operation, the female hormones—particularly estrogen—that keep the female body and brain functioning are no longer produced in the same amounts. In the absence of adequate quantities of estrogen, a woman may start to experience some of the following symptoms:

- anxiety
- backache
- depression
- difficulty sleeping
- discomfort or pain during intercourse
- dry skin
- dry vagina
- headaches
- hot flashes
- increased facial hair

❖ irritability

❖ itchy skin (as if insects are crawling on the skin)

❖ joint aches

❖ lack of sexual drive

❖ light-headedness

❖ loss of concentration

❖ mood swings

❖ muscle aches

❖ poor memory

❖ tiredness

❖ urinary stress incontinence

Menopausal symptoms often start a few years before a woman's periods stop altogether; during this time, referred to as *perimenopause,* the symptoms are at their most severe. Sometimes periods quit abruptly, but more commonly they are sporadic, wavering between heavy and light until they finally stop completely. When periods have ceased entirely for a year, a woman is said to have reached *menopause.* Symptoms vary from none to severe among individual women, and they may last from a few months to several years. The average age of menopause is around fifty, but it can range anywhere between ages thirty-five and fifty-nine.

Hot flashes are the most distressing symptom reported by women in Dr. Liew's practice. In mild cases, women report a wave of heat creeping up the trunk, neck, and face for a few minutes. Some also complain of severe sweating following a hot flash—this can occur twenty to thirty times a day. At night, these severely affected women have to change their pajamas or nightclothes a few times because of the sweats, and they are invariably unable to tolerate any blankets, whether it's summer or winter.

Another noted symptom is loss of libido (interest in sex), which can go hand in hand with dryness of the vagina, making intercourse uncomfortable and irritating. Often estrogen replacement alone is not enough to improve lack of sexual desire, but it definitely helps with vaginal lubrication, eases the symptoms of vaginitis, and decreases the risk of recurrent bladder infections. Plant estrogens, when eaten regularly for a few months, can help moisten a dry vagina, making sex more comfortable. Other symptoms, such as mood swings, irritability, and insomnia, may also respond quite well to estrogen supplementation.

Some complaints, although listed as symptoms of "menopause syndrome," may be the result of other medical conditions that are totally unrelated to menopause, but do occur more frequently in middle-aged and older people. These symptoms should be assessed and investigated on their merits, especially if they are distressing or disrupting your life. Two conditions that appear to affect middle-aged women more than other age groups are thyroid disorders and anemia.

⋙ Menopause and Hormone Replacement Therapy ⋘

Every woman (if she lives long enough) eventually goes through menopause. Some women sail through this phase of their lives without any problems, but a significant number require varying degrees of intervention and possibly even medical help with the multiple complaints associated with this time of life.

Hormone replacement therapy (HRT) may be the only answer for a certain number of women going through menopause. For these women, symptoms such as unbearable hot flashes and night sweats, an uncomfortably dry vagina, and roller-coaster mood swings may be alleviated only by HRT. For those whose lives have been drastically altered and their quality of life greatly diminished, medical treatment may indeed be the best option. There is no reason to suffer unduly during the menopausal years. Furthermore, it's well known that female hormones are inextricably linked to bone health, and thus HRT should be considered for those who are clearly at risk for osteoporosis. Recent research suggests that estrogen also enhances brain function and may be used to prevent and treat Alzheimer's disease in women. A large observational study carried out over the course of ten years in Cache County, Utah, reported that HRT use was associated with a significant reduction in the risk of Alzheimer's disease. At the time of the study, 72 percent of the study participants were using estrogens only while the rest were using combined

HRT. Other randomized clinical trials (RCT) of estrogens also reported varying improvement in the mental functions of treated participants. Unfortunately, these trials were small and short in duration. A large RCT that was designed to study the effects of estrogen (Premarin) on mental function and cognitive aging in postmenopausal women is expected to be completed in 2005.

On 28 May 2003, the authors from the Women's Health Initiative Memory Study reported that their randomized control trials of combined estrogen and progestin (Premarin and Prempo) had detected a two-fold increase in the risk of probable dementia (including Alzheimer's disease) in the HRT group when compared to the placebo group. This translates to an extra 23 cases of dementia per 10,000 women per year of HRT usage. It is not known if this increased risk is due to the progestin component of the HRT, as the results certainly contradicted those reported in previous observational studies and clinical trials.

Yet, the benefits of HRT may outweigh the risks for a number of women, in which case it should be seriously considered.

Benefits of HRT

- treats unbearable symptoms of menopause (hot flashes, dry vagina)
- preserves the bones and prevents osteoporosis
- may lower the risk for colon cancer
- has a questionable benefit in the prevention and treatment of Alzheimer's disease

But nothing works for everyone, and so it goes with HRT. Some women are unable to tolerate outside hormonal intervention in any form. It has been estimated that up to a third of women who start HRT discontinue it for one reason or another. (Recently, the WHI study reported a 42 percent discontinuation rate of the combined HRT.) One obvious reason for stopping treatment is the number of uncomfortable and unwanted side effects.

Common Side Effects of HRT

◈ fluid retention

◈ headaches

◈ irregular vaginal bleeding

◈ irritability

◈ nausea

◈ sore breasts

◈ venous thrombosis

◈ weight gain

A significant number of women simply cannot take HRT because it is contraindicated. This means that they currently have medical conditions that could be worsened by the addition of hormones. If you suffer from any of the following, HRT is not for you.

Contraindications of HRT

◈ deep venous thrombosis and/or pulmonary embolus

◈ endometriosis

◈ hormone-dependent cancers such as breast cancer, ovarian cancer, or endometrial (uterine) cancer

◈ impending surgery requiring immobilization

◈ liver disease

◈ undiagnosed vaginal bleeding

◈ uterine fibroids

Hormone replacement therapy during and after menopause greatly helps some women, but it's clearly not for everyone. Before you make the all-important decision to take or not take HRT, learn all you can about it, and know its risks as well as its benefits.

Potential Risks of HRT

◈ aggravation of preexisting hormone-dependent cancers

◈ deep venous thrombosis and/or pulmonary embolus

◈ increased risk of breast cancer

◈ increased risk of uterine cancer

◈ increased risk of coronary heart disease

◈ increased risk of stroke

In recent years, some menopause clinics have reported (in their observational studies) that HRT use by women after successful breast cancer therapy did not adversely affect their survival. Three clinical randomized trials to study the effects of HRT in patients with previous breast cancer are underway, but the results may not be available for quite some time yet. Until we are sure that HRT definitely will not cause harm to this group of women, the majority of doctors will probably not prescribe it for their breast cancer patients.

ᵐᵐ Plant Hormones Lessen Menopausal Symptoms ᵐᵐ

A lowered estrogen level is said to be responsible for many of the symptoms of menopause. While this is too simplistic an explanation for the entire anthology of menopause-related complaints, it is true that a number of disturbing feelings may accompany declining production of female hormones.

A host of researchers have noted that a common factor links women's diets in countries where women in midlife are free from menopause-related complaints. These women eat plant foods containing estrogen-like substances that augment natural estrogen in their bodies. Laboratory tests have also shown that estrogen-like substances in foods can, in fact, have a marked influence on women's hormone status and general health.

Certain plant foods, ingested in sufficient amounts, contain enough plant estrogens *(phytoestrogens)* to elevate hormonal levels and curtail menopausal symptoms. When estrogen levels are low, a daily dose of specific foods eaten at a meal or as a snack may provide just enough of a boost to ward off hot flashes, moisten vaginal tissue, and even out mood swings.

Food substances that simulate hormone activity in the body are called *phytohormones,* but in reality they aren't true hormones such as those produced naturally by our bodies. Phytohormones can affect estrogen activity directly, or they can provide precursors to substances that later promote estrogen activity. Phytohormones may have differing effects, depending on a woman's natural hormonal level at the time of ingestion. They can stimulate estrogen production if levels are too low, and they also can reduce hormone levels if they are too high. This property is referred to as *hormonal modulation,* and it is evident in herbs such as dong quai and panax ginseng. Phytoestrogens (particularly the subcategory known as *isoflavones*) compete with the body's natural estrogens by attaching themselves to estrogen receptor sites (alpha and beta) on cell surfaces when there are excessive amounts of estrogen in the body, thereby reducing the potent effect of naturally produced estrogens on sensitive tissues such as the breasts and uterus. In an estrogen-deficient state, when there are more empty estrogen receptor sites, phytoestrogens occupy the empty sites and behave like weak natural estrogens. Phytoestrogens can do this because their chemical structure closely resembles that of natural estrogens.

Literally hundreds of plants contain estrogen-like substances. Some foods contain more potent phytoestrogens than others. Studies have shown that soy, flaxseed, rye, clover, and chickpeas (garbanzo beans) are among those with the most potent hormonelike effects. The foods listed on page 18 contain one or more of the phytoestrogen groups, which are called *isoflavones, lignans,* and *coumestans.* (See the Appendix for a diagram illustrating how some of the different phytoestrogens are grouped in relation to each other.) This list is by no means complete; further research is being carried out all the time.

How Phytoestrogens React in a Woman's Body

How phytoestrogens work is still somewhat perplexing. They appear to have contradictory effects in women's bodies, depending on one's age and how much estrogen the body makes naturally. When a woman's estrogen levels wane, as in menopause, phytoestrogens exert estrogen-like activity and raise the estrogen level in the body's tissues; paradoxically, when a premenopausal woman generates high levels of estrogen, these same phytoestrogens block some of the natural estrogen from entering the cells, thus protecting against unhealthy exposure. Not only can phytoestrogens treat menopausal symptoms that result from declining estrogen levels, they also may protect against breast and uterine cancers, which are thought to be promoted by continuing exposure to high levels of estrogen.

It is thought that estrogen-like substances from plant sources bind to estrogen receptor sites within the body, thus reducing the effects of the low-estrogen state characteristic of menopause. Even though such proestrogenic activity is very weak (from $\frac{1}{400}$ to $\frac{1}{1,000}$ the strength of women's natural estrogen), the boost may be enough to circumvent symptoms.

Phytoestrogens' effect on female tissues depends on many factors: the two most obvious are the amount of estrogen a woman's body is already producing and the saturation of her receptor sites. If natural estrogen is sufficient or elevated, then phytoestrogens compete for status on the receptor sites. If they successfully replace the natural estrogen that our bodies make, they are thought to protect us from unhealthy levels of one type of estrogen, estradiol.

This information has helped to explain observational studies of post-menopausal Asian women, who have not only fewer menopausal symptoms but also a lower rate of breast cancer. Significant amounts of excreted phytoestrogen byproducts have been found in the urine of Asian women, from ten to one hundred times more than in that of Americans. Indeed, some researchers consider urinary excretion of plant estrogens a better indication of the health benefits such as reduction of cholesterol, blood pressure, and hot flashes than other types of laboratory tests. High urinary excretion of phytoestrogens suggests adequate consumption, bacterial transformation, and absorption of phytoestrogens. In other words, the amount of phytoestrogens present in the urine tends to predict how much you'll benefit from eating phytoestrogen-rich foods. (A minority of people, however, are unable to absorb or benefit from phytoestrogens despite eating large amounts of phytoestrogen-containing foods. These people are considered nonresponders.)

The Estrogen Food List

❖ LEGUMES ❖

alfalfa, black-eyed peas, black gram (mung beans), chickpeas (garbanzo beans), green or French beans, green peas, kidney beans, lentils, mung bean sprouts, navy beans, peanuts, red beans (adzuki beans), red clover, soybeans, soy sprouts, split or field peas

❖ OILS ❖

corn oil, flaxseed oil, olive oil, sesame oil, sunflower oil, rapeseed oil (canola oil)

❖ VEGETABLES ❖

beets, bok choy, broccoli, cabbage, carrots, cauliflower, celery, chives, cucumbers, eggplant, garlic, green peppers, mushrooms, onions, potatoes, pumpkin, radish, rhubarb, seaweed, squash, sweet potatoes, tomatoes, yams

❖ SPICES AND HERBS ❖

black cohosh, cloves, dong quai, fennel, ginger, hops, licorice, sage, tea, thyme, turmeric

❖ SEEDS AND NUTS ❖

anise seeds, caraway seeds, cashew nuts, flaxseeds, hazelnuts, pumpkin seeds, sesame seeds, sunflower seeds, walnuts

❖ FRUITS ❖

apples, avocados, black currants, cherries, cranberries, cantaloupe, gooseberries, grapes, guava, lemon, lychee, olives, oranges, papayas, pears, plums, pomegranates, prunes, raspberries, red currants, strawberries

❖ CEREALS/GRAINS ❖

barley, corn, oats, rice, rye, wheat

Studies on the incidence of breast, colon, and prostate cancers among Asians and residents of Western countries have suggested that the incidence of these cancers is linked to diet. Migrant Asian populations that adopt a Western diet—high in fats and low in vegetables and fiber—have a much higher incidence of these cancers than do the populations in their native lands. A typical Asian diet includes 30 to 100 milligrams of phytoestrogens daily; the Japanese consume up to 200 milligrams of phytoestrogens per day. Europeans and Americans take in a paltry 1 to 5 milligrams of phytoestrogens daily.

Properties of Soy Proteins

Phytoestrogens in general, but particularly those found in soy foods, contain specific hormonelike substances called *isoflavones*. This large class of compounds (there are well over four thousand) occurs naturally in plants and can be further subdivided into more specific types, including daidzein, genistein, formononetin, and biochanin A. One of these, *genistein,* is considered the most powerful within this class of isoflavones and seems to be generating the most interest among food scientists, especially for its role in cancer therapy. Many ongoing studies are evaluating exactly how it works in human health.

There is much to learn about isoflavones, but we know at this time that they are a prolific family with benefits that extend beyond boosting women's estrogen levels. Consider some of their varied properties:

- antibacterial
- antiviral
- antifungal
- anti-inflammatory
- antioxidant

These properties are important aids in our bodies' fight against harmful bacteria, viruses, and fungi, and thus isoflavone-containing foods help keep us in good health. Although our bodies call on the immune system and produce antibodies to fight invaders, we need all the help we can get, and natural foods help us stay in top shape. Isoflavones' antioxidant effects are especially beneficial when free radicals are overabundant in our bodies, causing the degeneration of body parts such as blood vessels and joints. Isoflavones, along with other antioxidants, wipe up the free radicals and thus prevent long-term damage to vital organs and systems.

Isoflavones are also thought to have the following effects:

◈ restricting the growth of tumors

◈ building bone

◈ lowering high blood pressure

◈ lowering total and low-density lipoprotein (LDL) cholesterol, otherwise known as "bad" cholesterol for its artery-clogging properties

◈ controlling hot flashes

It must be noted that although recent studies have shown that isoflavones can help preserve bone density, isoflavones are less effective in this regard than the estrogens used in HRT. Most of these studies were done on animals, and the majority of those that focused on humans were short term. However, in one study, whose results were reported in January 2001, Japanese researchers reported increased bone mass amongst postmenopausal women who had high consumption of soy products compared to those in the low-intake group. Results of other studies will hopefully confirm what population studies have already implied: that humans consuming large amounts of phytoestrogen-containing foods have lower osteoporotic fracture rates, thus emphasizing the osteoporosis-prevention effects of phytoestrogens.

Animal studies have shown that genistein in particular does inhibit bone breakdown in the body, thus maintaining the animals' bone density. Ipriflavone (a synthetic isoflavone) has been shown to maintain bone density in postmenopausal women, and it also slows bone density loss in women whose ovaries have been removed.

⌒ Studies on Soy and Hot Flashes ⌒

Is it possible that the natural estrogen diet will ever replace HRT as a way to curb menopausal symptoms? While the diet may not work for women with horrendous symptoms, there is evidence that it can effectively minimize hot flashes—among other symptoms—in moderate cases.

Isoflavones, which are found primarily in soy products, are basic to the Asian diet, and they are thought to be responsible for many health benefits specific to women. It has been estimated that the daily Asian diet may contain up to 50 grams of these soy proteins, as well as significant amounts of legumes, cereals, and grains, which are also rich in plant estrogens. Most experiments or trials use pure extracts of a particular isoflavone, but some studies have used or are now using soy flour or, more commonly, soy products to assess the effects of soy on blood pressure, cholesterol, hot flashes, and vaginal cell changes.

At the Second International Symposium on the Role of Soy in Preventing and Treating Chronic Disease (held in Brussels, Belgium, in September 1996), researchers looked at six human studies to determine the role of soy in reducing menopausal symptoms, especially hot flashes. While all six studies found at least a slight decline in the rate of hot flashes, three found a significant drop.

One of these studies, conducted in Melbourne, Australia, showed a 40 percent reduction in hot flashes when women consumed 40 grams of soy flour each day for twelve weeks. Similar results were found in the United Kingdom (using 80 grams of isoflavones for two months) and in Italy (using 60 milligrams of isolated soy protein with 76 milligrams of isoflavones).

Research in the U.S. from 1998 adds credence to the theory that phytoestrogens—specifically those found in soy—can ease menopausal hot flashes. In a double-blind, placebo-controlled study, over one hundred postmenopausal women, ages forty-eight to sixty-one, were divided into two groups. Each day for three months, each of the members of one group was given an inert nonsoy tablet (a placebo), and those in the other group were each given 60 grams of isolated soy protein. The number of hot flashes and night sweats experienced by the women getting the soy was reduced by 45 percent by the end of the twelve weeks, compared to 30 percent in the placebo group.

In March 2002 Spanish researchers found a 47.8 percent reduction in hot flashes amongst women using 17.5 milligrams of soy isoflavones twice daily for four months.

It must be noted that some studies of soy's effects find no significant relief from hot flashes when the treatment group is compared to the non-treatment group. This suggests several things. First, it suggests that the placebo effect is very strong; in other words, women in the nontreatment groups felt better simply because that was what they'd expected. Second, it suggests that some women may be more sensitive to soy than others; finally, it suggests that the dosages in some of the studies were inadequate to elicit a response. It is also possible that women in the nontreatment groups may have consumed foods containing other plant estrogens that had been overlooked in the studies.

How Much Soy Is Needed to Relieve Menopausal Symptoms?

No minimum daily requirement has been established for soy intake (or isoflavone content, as it is sometimes expressed). But the studies that have been conducted do provide clues as to what amount effectively reduces menopausal symptoms.

According to Loma Linda University soy pioneer and expert Mark Messina, Ph.D., the Japanese diet includes 30 to 50 milligrams of isoflavones on the average, which translates into about 10 to 25 grams of soy protein ingested per day. To help you convert figures between soy intake and isoflavone content, consider that soy products contain roughly 1 to 3 milligrams of isoflavones per gram of protein. To put this into more practical terms, one serving of soy contains, on average, between 4 and 12 grams of soy protein, or 12 to 45 milligrams of isoflavones.

A serving of soy is considered a half cup of tofu, tempeh, dry-roasted soy nuts, or green soybeans, or one cup of soy milk. The goal should be about 50 milligrams of isoflavones per day or two servings of soy, depending on the food's isoflavone content. We recommend that you not eat all the soy at one time; instead, spread it out among your meals and snacks.

The half-life of soy isoflavones is eight to twelve hours, meaning that the level of isoflavones in your blood drops by half within eight to twelve hours of ingesting the soy. Therefore, you'll get optimal results if you eat plant estrogens throughout the day.

It's not always easy to find out how much isoflavone is in the products you have chosen. Isoflavone levels in the soybean itself vary, and different brands of soy foods contain different levels of isoflavones, so there are wide discrepancies among otherwise similar foods. Many food companies now offer isoflavone content information on their packages, but due to these variables, you should recognize that the information may be inexact.

Many factors determine the phytoestrogen levels of soy foods and of other foods that we eat, and other variables determine how much phytoestrogen our bodies can absorb. These are outlined in the next section.

Factors Affecting Natural Phytoestrogens

- The season in which a plant is harvested is important in establishing its phytoestrogen content. Asians traditionally have been fussy about the timing of the harvest of plant and animal products. This knowledge is passed on from generation to generation, even though it is not generally accompanied by a scientific explanation. It is now known that concentrations of phytoestrogens vary with the maturity of the plant and the timing of its harvest.

- The genetic origin of the plant, and the climatic and environmental conditions under which it grew, also affect its phytoestrogen levels. For example, drought causes plants' phytoestrogen concentrations to increase. Genetic alteration of plants such as soy also affects phytoestrogen content.

- Processing of plant foods also affects phytoestrogen levels—the more a plant is processed, the lower its phytoestrogen content.

Even if a plant food's phytoestrogen levels are high, individual factors may affect how well the phytoestrogens are absorbed by our bodies:

◈ Appropriate bacteria must be present in the intestine of the consumer in order to properly digest and absorb phytoestrogens.

◈ The transit time of the plant product in the intestine determines how much phytoestrogen can be absorbed. Absorption depends on a normal and efficient gastrointestinal system.

Other Natural Remedies That Regulate Hormonal Status

We can minimize the transitory symptoms of menopause by simply changing our dietary and lifestyle habits. These changes include incorporating soy and other phytoestrogen-rich foods into our diets, but there are other steps we can take as well. Following are some of the suggestions outlined in Linda Ojeda's book *Menopause Without Medicine*.

◈ A **high-fiber diet** promotes the excretion of estrogen. Some women produce too much estrogen, and thus are at risk for estrogen-based cancers. A diet that includes 20 to 40 grams of fiber a day includes enough fiber so that some will bind with estrogen in the intestinal tract and help remove it from the body.

◈ **Bioflavonoids** are compounds with structural and chemical similarities to estrogen, and they help to regulate estrogen levels in much the same way as phytoestrogens. They have been shown to control hot flashes, mood swings, anxiety, and heavy menstrual bleeding. Bioflavonoids are found in citrus fruits, grapes, cherries, cantaloupe, tomatoes, green peppers, and rose hips.

◈ A **low-fat diet**, with fat between 25 and 30 percent of total caloric intake, limits production of estrogen and encourages the excretion of excess estrogen.

◈ **Vitamin E**, which is essential for the production of sex hormones, effectively reduces menopausal symptoms such as hot flashes, vaginal dryness, and mood swings, and protects against heart disease and cancer. It's found in oil, nuts, seeds, sweet potatoes, and wheat germ. Results are more effective with supplements in doses between 100 and 400 IU (international units), because the amount of vitamin E we receive from food is inadequate to minimize symptoms or protect us from heart disease and cancer.

❧ The essential fatty acids found in **flaxseed** act as weak estrogens in the body and thus help to keep all the tissues in the body well lubricated, including the skin, hair, and vaginal lining. These essential fats have been shown to reduce symptoms of menopause if they are ingested in doses of 25 grams (one to two tablespoons) per day.

❧ **B vitamins** are instrumental in regulating estrogen in the body. When the Bs are insufficient, estrogen levels escalate. B vitamins are found in whole grains, beans, peas, chicken, and beef.

❧ **Boron** can mimic and enhance the action of estrogen and is needed to aid in calcium metabolism. Boron is found abundantly in fruits and vegetables, nuts, and flaxseed.

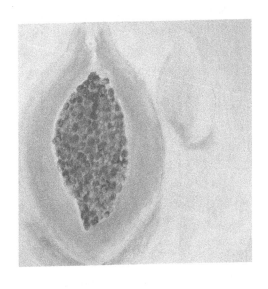

Chapter Two

Plant Hormones &
Other Health Concerns
for Women

U p to this point in the book, we've been discussing the ways in which we can augment falling estrogen levels in menopause in order to stave off uncomfortable symptoms and possibly protect ourselves from heart disease and cancer. However, it's important to note that while most menopausal women experience declining estrogen levels, some *premenopausal* women are far from deficient in this female hormone. In fact, many women make more estrogen than they need. This may be due to heredity or to diet and lifestyle.

Over a lifetime, overexposure to estrogen can contribute to estrogen-based cancers of the breast and uterus. This chapter explains how phytoestrogen-containing foods may help to fend off such cancers and also details the other, numerous benefits that these foods can offer both premenopausal and menopausal women. Hopefully, women who have not yet reached menopause will be open to dietary and lifestyle changes that can benefit their future health.

How Phytoestrogens Protect Against Breast Cancer

There is strong epidemiological evidence that diet plays a role in the development of breast cancer. This hypothesis was derived from population and migration studies that observed the food selections of various cultures throughout the world. The bulk of this research pointed to a high-fat diet as the culprit predisposing a woman to breast cancer; however, when the results of a large study failed to support that hypothesis, interest began to focus upon other dietary factors.

Phytoestrogens are presently grabbing the attention of scientists and researchers around the world because diets containing high amounts of specific phytohormones have been correlated with a substantial reduction in breast cancer risk. For example, in a case-controlled study of more than six hundred premenopausal women in Singapore, it was found that those who consumed the most soy were less likely to develop breast cancer than those who rarely touched it. Soy, the major source of isoflavones, seems to lengthen the menstrual cycle by one to five days, thus reducing the cells' exposure to estrogen and cutting the risk of breast cancer. Asian women are known to have longer menstrual cycles than Western women, as well as a lower risk of breast cancer.

Another case-control study, conducted in Australia by David Ingram, M.D., and published in the *Lancet* in 1997, likewise found an association between phytoestrogen intake (as measured by urinary excretion) and the risk of breast cancer. After adjusting for possible confounding factors, such as age, parity (whether a woman has had children, and how many she has had), and alcohol and fat intake, the researchers noted a substantial reduction in breast cancer risk. This reduction, they felt, was unlikely to result from mere chance.

It is generally accepted that when estrogen levels stay too elevated for too long, a woman's risk of breast cancer increases. Reducing the effect of estrogen, it is widely believed, can produce a four- to five-fold reduction in breast cancer. One way to curtail estrogen production is to block the body's estrogen receptors before they can be filled with the strongest form of estrogen, estradiol. Specific isoflavones in soy, those called *genistein* and *daidzein,* attach to the receptors in the breast and block estradiol, which is known to stimulate cancer cells in the breast. Two popular anticancer prescription drugs, tamoxifen and raloxifene, work the same way, although tamoxifen stimulates uterine cells at the same time; phytoestrogens do not adversely affect uterine cells. Indeed, plant estrogens appear to exert a positive influence on uterine cells, and thus foods containing phytoestrogens have been studied in relation to another frightening female cancer, uterine cancer. Mark Goodman and his team at the Cancer Research Center of Hawaii studied 332 women of many different ethnic backgrounds and compared them to a control group. At the end of the study, the researchers found that the women who ate the most phytoestrogen-rich foods, including tofu and beans, had a 54 percent reduction in the risk of uterine cancer.

Soy and flaxseed, another phytoestrogen-rich food, contain yet another family of plant components, called *lignans,* that are thought to reduce both estrogen exposure and cancer risk. Lignans are a type of fiber that is changed by friendly bacteria in the gut into compounds that fight against cancer. Lignans have a biochemical structure similar to that of isoflavones and women's own natural estrogen, and thus they are able to fill estrogen receptors and thwart normal estrogen activity. Studies have shown that women who have breast cancer excrete lower amounts of lignans than do healthy women.

Lignans are structural components of plants such as fruits, legumes, vegetables, and grains, but they are found in greatest concentration in flaxseed (not the oil, just the seeds). The National Cancer Institute is looking at flaxseed as a potential cancer-fighter because it houses both lignans and omega-3 fatty acids, a healthy type of fat that shrinks cancer tumors and has a potent effect on breast, prostate, and lung cancer cells.

No one is saying that soy and flaxseed alone are going to cut your risk of cancer. But evidence suggests that one or two daily portions of soy and a tablespoon of flaxseed, along with other cancer-fighting nutrients and lifestyle changes, may reduce your risk. Since such a regimen causes no harm to the body—and indeed brings benefits—and since there is at least a chance that it might reduce your cancer risk, why not give it a try?

Other Ways to Slow Down Estrogen Production in the Breast

Pay Attention to the Kinds of Fat You Eat

The kind of fat you eat is more important than the amount of fat in your diet. A classic study of 350,000 women in 1996, reported in the *New England Journal of Medicine,* debunked the theory that a high-fat diet increased the risk of breast cancer. After one sifts through the research, it becomes clear that the types of fat, rather than merely the amount of fat, that women eat can possibly promote or prevent breast cancer.

Fats to Avoid

Saturated fats—found in red meats and whole-fat dairy products like milk, butter, cheese, and creams

Trans fatty acids—found in many margarines, fried foods, crackers, cookies, and bakery products (look for the phrase **partially hydrogenated vegetable oil** in the ingredient list, and avoid products that contain it)

Polyunsaturated oils—safflower oil, corn oil, soybean oil, peanut oil, and sesame oil

According to the current scientific literature, the safest oils are believed to be olive oil and canola oil, two monounsaturated oils. A recent Swedish study of over sixty thousand women reported that monounsaturated fat reduced the risk of breast cancer by 45 percent. Two tablespoons per day in place of other fats is recommended.

Oils from fresh fish are an easy way to cut down on the body's excess estrogen. The omega-3 fatty acids found in cold-water fish (such as salmon, mackerel, and herring) and in cod liver oil have actually reduced tumors in lab tests and in studies on animals and humans. Many scientific journals have published accounts of omega-3 fatty acids being used in supplement form to treat various cancers. Don't overdo it; unless you are under the care of a physician, we do not advise megadosing with any supplement, including omega-3 fatty acids. However, choosing fish for dinner a few times a week and using olive or canola oil in your cooking are safe ways to provide the healthy fats your body needs.

Maintain a High-Fiber Diet

A diet that includes plenty of fiber enhances excretion of estrogen from the body. One study showed that Finnish women who ate a high-fat diet but also incorporated adequate daily fiber had two-thirds the incidence of breast cancer of Western women.

Fiber may also bind with and dispose of carcinogens that we ingest in foods and absorb from the environment, making it doubly protective. Women who eat whole grains, beans, fruits, and vegetables are rarely constipated, and it appears that there is a relationship between constipation and breast cancer. Women who have two or fewer bowel movements per week experience four times the incidence of breast cancer of women who have a bowel movement once a day.

Recommended daily fiber amounts range between 30 and 40 grams. High-fiber cereals and legumes are your best sources.

Keep Your Body Fat Moderate to Low

Excess body fat means excess estrogen. Body fat encourages estrogen production, and too much estrogen makes it very easy for the body to store fat, and thus a vicious cycle begins. If you are already overweight, it is not easy to stop this cycle, especially if you are older and if you have dieted and regained your weight several times. Losing weight slowly through exercise and limiting calories (particularly by avoiding large amounts of carbohydrates—sugars and starches—at one sitting) works for most women. Whatever you do, avoid an ultra-low-fat diet. (In other words, don't let your fat intake fall below 15 percent of your daily calories. The optimal level of fat intake is between 20 percent and 30 percent of total calories.) Such diets are ineffective for most women, and they rob you of essential fats and fat-soluble vitamins.

Try Cruciferous Vegetables

Vegetables from the cabbage family—which includes cabbage, broccoli, bok choy, Brussels sprouts, cauliflower, kale, turnips, radishes, and watercress—play a role in curtailing the formation of cancer cells. An ingredient called *indole-3-carbinol* turns estrogen into another substance less harmful to the body. Also found in such vegetables are many sulfur-containing compounds; one class of these compounds, called *glucosinolates,* has also shown anticancer properties.

Be Cautious with Alcohol

Alcohol causes estrogen levels to rise. Even light to moderate drinking slows down the burning of fats, making it easy to store fat on the body. Couple drinking with eating high-fat foods, and you have a recipe for obesity. If you are already overweight (and thus overproduce natural estrogen), alcohol may have an even more damaging effect. Heavy drinkers (women who drink more than four glasses of alcohol per day) increase their chances of getting breast cancer by more than 40 percent and hip fractures by nearly two and a half times.

⌇ Women, Heart Disease, and HRT ⌇

Most women fear breast cancer more than heart disease, yet nearly twice as many women die from heart disease and stroke than from all forms of cancer combined. Although 2.5 million American women are hospitalized for cardiovascular disease each year (of these, five hundred thousand die), women remain in the dark about what is taking their lives.

Women may fail to realize that heart disease is a different experience for women than for men. Women are less likely than men to be diagnosed with heart disease, and women are less likely to recover from it. Medications and medical interventions that save men's lives may be less effective for women. Even the diet that has been proposed as the standard heart diet may be inappropriate for women. (For the full report on women and heart disease, read *Her Healthy Heart,* by Linda Ojeda.)

In the past, one of HRT's major marketing claims was that it protected against heart disease. But in light of recent studies, that benefit can no longer be claimed.

A landmark study, the Heart and Estrogen-Progestin Replacement Study (HERS), found that postmenopausal women with existing coronary heart disease received no benefit from HRT. This study, which was the first randomized, controlled trial of HRT, was published in the *Journal of the American Medical Association* on 19 August 1998. The researchers recommended that women with coronary heart disease should *not* take HRT solely as a hedge against heart disease. The study also confirmed earlier findings that the hormone preparation produced higher rates of gallbladder disease, increased blood clotting in the legs and lungs, and raised levels of triglycerides (a type of unhealthy fat that can harm the heart).

More alarming news was released on 17 July 2002 by the investigators of the WHI (Women's Health Initiative) study. This randomized, placebo-controlled study found a 29 percent *increase* in coronary heart disease amongst healthy postmenopausal women taking combined HRT compared to the group who was taking the inactive treatment (placebo). Cardiologists are certainly echoing the researchers' concern and now warn against the use of HRT for the prevention of heart disease.

Soy Protects the Heart

Incorporating soy into your diet may be a preferable alternative to HRT. Eight decades of accumulated evidence indicates that soy protein significantly affects blood cholesterol and strengthens the heart in several ways. An exhaustive meta-analysis of thirty-eight studies examining the effect of soy protein on serum lipid (blood fat) levels showed the following average reductions in cholesterol:

◈ Total cholesterol declined by 23.2 mg/dl★ (9.3 percent).

◈ LDL cholesterol dropped by 21.7 mg/dl★ (12.9 percent).

◈ Triglycerides declined by 13.3 mg/dl★ (10.5 percent).

★milligrams per deciliter

The authors of this comprehensive review of the literature stated that soy can reduce the risk of coronary heart disease by 18 to 28 percent. Specifically, their analysis indicated the following:

◈ A daily intake of 25 grams of soy protein over several months could reduce blood cholesterol by 8.9 mg/dl.

◈ An intake of 50 grams of soy protein could reduce it by 17.4 mg/dl.

◈ An intake of 75 grams could reduce it by 26.3 mg/dl.

If a low-fat diet has failed to lower your cholesterol levels, try soy. In a study at the University of Illinois, sixty-six postmenopausal women with cholesterol readings above 200 mg/dl were divided into two groups. Half followed a low-fat diet, using nonfat milk as the protein source, and the other half were given soy. Both groups experienced a reduction in total cholesterol; however, only the soy group saw a significant reduction in LDLs (low-density lipoproteins, the so-called bad cholesterol) plus a rise in HDLs (high-density lipoproteins, the so-called good cholesterol. See the glossary in the back of the book for more discussion of these two terms). However, the researchers noted that such results were seen in women with high cholesterol levels. If your cholesterol levels are within the average range, you probably won't notice any change.

After assessing more than fifty human trials conducted to study the effects of soy on blood lipid levels, the United States FDA approved the use of a soy health claim in the labeling of soy protein–containing foods. The approved label reads, "25 grams of soy protein a day, as part of a diet low in saturated fat and cholesterol, may reduce the risk of heart disease."

Soy proteins have several antiatherogenic (heart-healthy) effects in addition to lowering cholesterol. Consider the following:

◈ Soy isoflavones, phytates, and saponins have strong antioxidant activity and help curb the formation of toxic free radicals, which contribute to arterial damage.

◈ There is some evidence that genistein, the principal phyto-estrogen in soy, may work in the early stages of atherosclerosis (a condition that leads to clogged arteries, diminished blood flow, and possible heart failure) by hindering the overgrowth of epithelial cells lining the arteries. Such overgrowth promotes plaque buildup and clogged arteries.

◈ Genistein also appears to prevent blood clots, which can lead to heart attack and stroke, by inhibiting the formation of an enzyme called *thrombin*.

◈ Genistein may increase the flexibility of blood vessels, helping to prevent spasms that can trigger a heart attack.

◈ Soy has a modulating effect on blood sugar levels. Glycine and arginine, the amino acids in soy, decrease insulin levels in the blood, thus tempering blood sugar levels. Keeping blood sugar fairly stable is important for women, because the combination of high estrogen levels and high insulin levels has a doubly negative effect on both the heart and the breasts.

Other Heart-Healthy Strategies

◈ Cut down or eliminate saturated fats (found in red meats and whole-fat dairy products), trans fatty acids (found in many margarines, hydrogenated bakery products, and fried foods), and polyunsaturated oils (safflower, corn, and sunflower oils). All three negatively affect blood cholesterol levels and make women more vulnerable to heart disease.

◈ Fats that hold the stamp of approval include the monounsaturated oils, olive and canola. They have potent antioxidant properties that fend off artery damage from LDL cholesterol, and they've been shown to reduce LDLs without lowering HDLs.

The marine omega-3 fatty acids (which are found in certain fish) show great promise for keeping hearts healthy. A study at the University of Washington, which looked at both women and men, found that those who reported eating one serving of fatty fish a week had half the risk of heart attacks of those who shunned fish.

❖ Don't go too low with your fats. In a report in the 1 September 1998 issue of *Circulation,* the American Heart Association stated that very-low-fat diets may not provide additional benefits for the heart. The report, which summarized several clinical studies, indicated that cutting fat to less than 15 percent of total daily calories may lower beneficial HDLs and raise triglycerides, changes that are thought to raise heart disease risk. The optimal level of fat intake for heart health is between 20 and 30 percent of total calories.

❖ Soluble fiber, as found in oat bran, beans, legumes, apples, carrots, and whole grains, promotes the excretion of cholesterol and lowers both total and LDL cholesterol. It improves sugar metabolism, reduces blood insulin levels, and delays the emptying of the stomach, producing a feeling of fullness that can be useful if you wish to lose weight.

According to the Harvard School of Public Health, omitting fiber from the diet is just as important a risk factor for heart disease as cigarette smoking, high blood cholesterol, and high blood pressure. Your total daily fiber goal should be 30 to 40 grams; of that, one-third of the total (12 grams) should be soluble fiber. Sources of soluble fiber are listed below.

Sources of soluble fiber: 2–3 grams

Up to 1 cup bran and oat cereals (depending on brand)
$\frac{1}{2}$ cup cooked kidney beans
1 large apple
$\frac{1}{2}$ cup Brussels sprouts

Sources of soluble fiber: about 1 gram

Up to 1 cup other cereals
$\frac{1}{2}$ cup cooked split peas
1 carrot
3 dried prunes
$\frac{3}{4}$ cup asparagus

⬧ Flaxseed lowers cholesterol. It is also the primary source of healthy omega-3 fatty acids in the plant kingdom. While flaxseed oil is less potent than the fat of cold-water fish, it does provide unique benefits that set it apart and establish it as a superb fat for the heart. Another essential fatty acid (EFA) found in flaxseed, alpha linolenic acid, may protect against stroke. This particular EFA can reduce the "stickiness" of the blood's platelets, thus preventing dangerous blood clots from forming. Flaxseed is also a fair source of both soluble and insoluble fiber (an eighth of a cup offers 10 grams of fiber). It houses lignan precursors that are converted by bacteria during digestion into phytoestrogens. Because of any one or all of these factors, flaxseed has been shown to lower cholesterol between 5 and 15 percent. Various studies on flaxseed have used daily amounts between 5 and 50 grams to effect changes in blood fats.

⬧ An array of antioxidants, such as vitamins C and E, beta-carotene, and a host of others, guard against heart disease by preventing LDL cholesterol from oxidation by free radicals. Although the list of studies on the benefits of individual antioxidants seems endless, an important study out of Harvard University has demonstrated that these potent health-protecting nutrients work best in combination. Women who took vitamin E and C and beta-carotene on a regular basis experienced a remarkable decrease in heart disease risk—50 percent—and their stroke rate fell by 54 percent.

To get a healthy dose of antioxidants, we should eat two to three servings of fruit and four to five servings of vegetables per day. Because few people manage to eat the requisite number of servings, a multivitamin/mineral tablet taken as a supplement may be necessary. Note that supplements should be used as an adjunct to these wonderful fruits and vegetables, not as a replacement for them.

❖ Getting enough of three B vitamins—folic acid and vitamins B-6 and B-12—should be a major concern for anyone at risk for heart disease. When any one of the trio is lacking, homo-cysteine levels may rise in the blood. Homocysteine is a normal substance in the blood, but when it is elevated, it is considered one of the top risk factors for heart disease. In July 1997, *The New England Journal of Medicine* uncovered more than seventy-five clinical and observational studies that demonstrated a relationship between high homocysteine levels and coronary artery disease, peripheral artery disease, and stroke.

Researchers from the Harvard School of Public Health have proposed the theory that homocysteine damages the arteries' inner lining, beginning a process that fosters the proliferation of epithelial cells and plaque buildup. Other researchers have suggested that homocysteine seems to thicken the blood and may also facilitate the oxidation of LDL cholesterol.

Menopausal women are particularly at risk, because when estrogen wanes, homocysteine rises. To ensure that you get 400 micrograms of folic acid each day, breakfast on a bowl of folic acid–fortified cereal, lunch on a bowl of lentils, and snack on a variety of fruits and vegetables. If this doesn't sound doable, consider taking multivitamin and mineral tablets, which offer the requisite amount of folic acid as well as moderate amounts of vitamins B-6 and B-12. We recommend a vitamin tablet containing between 20 and 50 micrograms of both vitamins B-6 and B-12.

❖ Garlic has been reported to lower total cholesterol by 15 to 20 percent, to lower LDLs and triglycerides, and to increase HDLs.

It reduces blood pressure and blunts the blood's clotting tendency (clotting can lead to heart attacks). Incorporating garlic into your cooking, using it as an accompaniment to vegetable dishes, or offering it as an appetizer, along with the other dietary guidelines outlined in this book, may ward off a heart attack as well as any lurking vampires.

◈ Modern science has confirmed what early Egyptian writings noted about onions: they are a tonic for the blood. Scientific literature has reported that onions inhibit the formation of fibrinogen, which is a substance that the body produces to ensure proper blood clotting, especially when injury occurs. Thus onions can help to break up and dissolve potentially dangerous clots. Harvard cardiologist Victor Gurewich, M.D., found in his practice that taking the juice of a single onion daily raised HDL levels about 70 percent of the time.

◈ Green tea possesses important polyphenols, which are yet another group of phytochemicals that possess potent antioxidant properties. Substitute green tea for your morning coffee or late afternoon pick-me-up.

Hormones Prevent Bone Loss

It is well known that both estrogen and progesterone help preserve women's bone density, and as a result millions of American women take HRT to protect against bone loss, which leads to osteoporosis. Estrogen prevents the bone loss that accompanies menopause. It does not reverse already established osteoporosis, but it does stop natural or accelerated bone deterioration. Doctors were recommending that HRT be continued indefinitely to be successful. However, subsequent to the data from the WHI study (released in July 2002), bone specialists are revising their advice regarding long-term combined HRT use by their female patients. Although the study confirmed the reduction of hip, vertebral, and other fractures in women taking HRT, the increased risks for breast cancer, coronary artery disease (CAD), strokes, deep-vein thrombosis (DVT), and lung clots are too much a trade off to a healthy woman.

Low-dose estrogen preparations (0.3 milligrams) have been found to be as effective in preventing bone loss as the standard 0.625-milligram formulation. It's quite possible that a lower dosage also causes fewer side effects, so it may be tolerable for women who were forced to discontinue their treatment due to uncomfortable side effects. It is still unknown whether a lower dosage lessens the risk for breast cancer, CAD, strokes, and the like. The arm of the WHI study that reported a 26 percent increase in breast cancer rates used the 0.625-milligram dose of conjugated equine estrogens (Premarin).

Some studies suggest that progesterone is the more important female hormone in the battle against osteoporosis because it actually builds new bone. In what is now called a landmark study of progesterone, John Lee, M.D., asked postmenopausal women with existing osteoporosis to apply a cream containing 3 percent progesterone to their skin for two weeks out of the month. He also advised them to follow specific dietary guidelines and take nutritional supplements. The study found that, among one hundred patients who had serious bone loss, sixty-three experienced bone-density increases of 15.4 percent following the treatment. The expected bone-density loss for this age group is 4.5 percent.

Natural progesterone, as opposed to the synthetic progestins found in oral preparations, appears to be relatively free of side effects. Conclusive research has yet to be done, but many nutritionally oriented doctors are prescribing natural progesterone, and an even larger number of women are utilizing this approach. It is generally recommended that women apply one-quarter to one-half teaspoon of progesterone cream to their inner arms, abdomen, or inner thighs for two weeks out of the month and that they rotate the sites of cream application. Because many of the natural-progesterone products on the market contain very small amounts of the hormone, this book's Resources section lists a few that are reputable and contain known quantities of the hormone. You can also get information about these creams and their use from their manufacturers.

Can Plant Hormones Protect Bones?

Researchers have still not determined with absolute certainty whether plant hormones are potent enough to prevent or arrest bone loss. It is known that the isoflavones genistein and daidzein are similar to synthetic estrogen, which is effective in preventing or retarding bone loss, but whether they can replace HRT is not yet known.

Early research found that isoflavones had a modest effect on bone tissue, but more recent studies appear more encouraging. Research conducted by John Anderson, of the University of North Carolina, showed that soy protein did prevent bone deterioration in rats whose ovaries had been removed, resulting in a diminished estrogen supply and attendant bone loss. When this group of rodents was compared to another group taking Premarin (the most common HRT medication, made from the urine of pregnant mares), the results showed that soy could prevent bone loss almost as well as synthetic hormones.

In a study on postmenopausal women, researchers from the University of Illinois compared sixty-six women who drank milk protein to a group of women who received soy protein that contained either 56 or 90 milligrams of isoflavones. The women who took soy protein with 90 milligrams of isoflavones every day for six months were found to have higher bone mineral density in their spines. Researcher Susan Potter found this encouraging but pointed out that the studies need to be extended over one to three years. The study also found that doses of isoflavones below 90 milligrams did not work.

A review covering published reports on population studies, lab cultures on cells and tissues, and experimental studies on animals concluded that taking isoflavones (especially genistein and daidzein) at optimal doses resulted in improved bone mass.

How much isoflavone should you take to treat and prevent bone loss? Experts have speculatively suggested that between 16 and 20 grams of soy protein (which would provide 16 to 60 milligrams of isoflavone) taken daily is sufficient for prevention. Practically, for those of us who think in terms of servings of a food, this means one to two servings of soy per day. For treatment, the studies used 90 milligrams of isoflavones, which means that you would have to double the servings of soy per day. Many women may find this impractical and would rather take their chances with HRT. However, other options are available; these are discussed on the following page.

A synthetic isoflavone called *ipriflavone,* in a dosage of 200 milligrams taken three times per day, has been found by various researchers to preserve bone mineral density. All these studies were small and ran for up to two years duration. A larger European study that ran for three years failed to show any significant changes in bone mineral density between the treated and placebo groups. Furthermore, the authors found lower lymphocyte (a type of white blood cell) counts in the treated group, potentially problematic because of white blood cells' important role in the health of the immune system.

In September 1999, at the North American Menopause Society meeting in New York, Sydney researcher Dr. R. Baber and his colleagues presented their findings regarding a red-clover extract, marketed under the brand name Rimostil, which contains 57 milligrams of isoflavones. They reported a significant increase in the bone density of the forearm bones after just six months of treatment with Rimostil. More importantly, when they checked the uterus, they found no significant changes in the thickness of the lining. The bonuses reported from this study included improvement in the lipids profile and absence of uterine bleeding.

In addition, drugs such as raloxifene (Evista), alendronate (Fosamax), and risedronate (Actonel) are currently available for the treatment of osteoporosis. They are not without side effects, however, so discuss them with your doctor.

If you are determined to use natural methods to prevent osteoporosis but cannot incorporate the recommended amount of soy in your diet, don't get discouraged. Remember that soy is but one of many ways to keep the bones healthy. In fact, we should all remember that soy foods and medication should be combined with other bone-building practices in order to be effective. The next section outlines some of these practices.

✎ A Lifestyle Program to Build Bones ✎

Soy and other estrogen-rich foods may spare you further bone loss, so it makes sense to include these foods in your anti-osteoporosis diet. However, a complete bone-healthy program should also include the following:

❧ Stop smoking. Female smokers lose bone mass faster than non-smokers, probably because the associated drop in estrogen may diminish absorption of calcium.

❧ Limit caffeine. Excess intake is associated with increased urinary excretion of calcium.

❧ Limit sodas. They are high in phosphoric acid, which interferes with your intestinal calcium absorption and urinary excretion.

❧ Your basic diet should be high in carbohydrates, relatively low in fat, and low in meat proteins. Red meat is very high in phosphorus, a mineral that in high doses leaches calcium from the bones.

❧ Keep your alcohol intake moderate. Too much alcohol causes calcium to be poorly absorbed and interferes with vitamin D metabolism.

❧ Make certain you get the full supply of bone-building nutrients, discussed below:

> *Calcium* is critical to bone health. The National Institutes of Health suggest that women up to age fifty, as well as postmenopausal women on HRT, should get 1,000 milligrams daily. For postmenopausal women not on HRT, 1,500 milligrams is recommended. Good food sources include low-fat yogurt and milk, tofu made with calcium sulfate, almonds, fortified cereals, and leafy green vegetables.

> *Magnesium* deficiency may weaken bones as much as inadequate calcium. A study at Purdue University found that menopausal women given magnesium hydroxide for two years saw a significant increase in bone density. Your daily magnesium intake should be between 500 and 800 milligrams per day. Dietary surveys have shown that up to 85 percent of American women consume less than the recommended daily allowance (RDA).

> *Vitamin D,* the sunshine vitamin, is needed to absorb calcium. Women should take in about 400 IU (international units) per

day. A thirty-minute walk in the sun, if your skin is exposed, provides about 300 IU.

Boron, the mineral found in nuts, beans, fruits, and vegetables, helps raise levels of blood estrogens in postmenopausal women, which may help them to retain calcium. Taking a 3-milligram boron supplement daily has been shown to reduce calcium excretion by 44 percent. If you regularly eat your fruits and veggies, supplements aren't necessary.

Many other nutrients affect calcium absorption and bone health. Consider some of the lesser-known vitamins and minerals that protect the bones: vitamins C and K, and the minerals manganese and copper.

◈ Exercise. Bone density depends on how much the bone is stressed. Women on estrogen who do not exercise do not gain bone mass. Weight-bearing exercises such as walking, dancing, and weight training, done for thirty minutes three times a week, strengthen your bones, heart, and entire body.

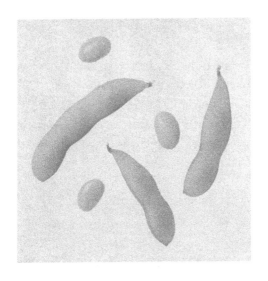

Chapter Three

An
Introduction
to *Soy*

ot too long ago, soy products were found only in Asian markets and health-food stores, but given their glowing promise for a variety of health concerns, they are worming their way onto the shelves of local supermarkets. Once nondescript oddities, soy products are now manufactured with American tastes in mind, and the variety of soy-based foods is expanding every year. Still, habits are slow to change, and we are often reluctant to try foods that have been foreign to our diets for so long. This chapter will introduce you to the ever-increasing choices in soy, but before we begin, it is important to understand why soy is considered such a superb food and why we encourage you to make it a regular part of your diet.

Nutritional Content of Soy

Soy is loaded with nutrition. It's what nutritionists call a nutrient-dense food. Soy is a complete protein; in fact, it's the only vegetable food that earns this title. It is higher in protein than other legumes, weighing in at 35 percent (in contrast to the 20 to 30 percent protein content of most other beans). Soy is high in complex carbohydrates and is a good source of both kinds of fiber (soluble and insoluble).

While soy can be high in fat (sometimes containing up to 40 percent fat), it is low in saturated fat. The predominant fat in soy is the essential fatty acid linoleic acid, an omega-6 fatty acid. But soy also contains some of the super-healthy omega-3 fatty acids. Not all soy products are high-fat. For example, texturized vegetable protein (TVP) has no fat, and many products are now manufactured with a lower fat content.

Soy is a good source of B vitamins, several micronutrients, and phytochemicals. It is a concentrated source of isoflavones, containing about 1 to 3 milligrams of isoflavones per gram of protein.

The Many Faces of Soy

See Chapter 4 for detailed information on the protein, fat, and caloric content of soy foods.

Soybeans

Soybeans belong to the legume family. The plant produces pods that, when mature, each contain two or three seeds. These seeds are the famous soybeans—sometimes called *soya beans*—which have been used in China for several thousand years. In China, the soybean is commonly known as *wang tul* or "yellow bean."

Dried soybeans are a yellowish to creamy color with a rather tough skin, and they're slightly smaller in size than green or garden peas. Soybeans can be purchased dried, like other beans, or fresh, as green soybeans. Either way, they contain about 35 percent protein by weight and are a good source of isoflavones, B vitamins, calcium, and fiber. The downside is that soybeans are harder to find than some of the other soy products, and they are decidedly tougher than most other types of beans. Many people find the flavor on the strong side; so if it is not to your liking, choose other soy foods.

Dried soybeans can be boiled for several hours, like any other bean, and eaten as a side dish or added to salads or casseroles. Fresh green soybeans look like fuzzy green pods. When they are steamed until tender, they are sweet and crunchy and are a great addition to salads or can be eaten plain as a snack. Soybeans in the pod, known as *edamame,* a standard Japanese snack, can be found in stores, already cooked and ready to eat, or frozen and needing to be boiled for a few minutes. Canned soybeans are also available. They can be easily served on toast or mixed into salads or casseroles.

Soy Milk and Other Soy Drinks

Soy milk is a milklike liquid prepared from ground soybeans and water. It is lactose-free, and people who cannot digest the sugar in cow's milk often drink it as a substitute. Unfortified soy milk is packed with protein (about 8 grams per cup, although this varies), B vitamins, and isoflavones. It contains less calcium than cow's milk, but like cow's milk it may be fortified with calcium, vitamin D, and sometimes vitamin B-12.

Manufacturers have made great strides in making soy milk palatable. No longer is it the grainy, beany drink of the past. Today, soy milk is light and smooth, and it is sold plain and in a variety of flavors, including chocolate, almond, and vanilla. You can find it next to "real" milk in the refrigerated section of the market, or you can buy it packaged in aseptic quart containers or snack sizes that do not need refrigeration. Soy milk is also available in low-fat and nonfat varieties.

Soy milk is good enough to drink hot or cold; you can pour it over cereal or use it as a milk substitute in cooking.

Soy Nuts

Soy nuts are dry-roasted or deep-fried soybeans that are normally flavored with salt or other seasonings. They're quick and tasty snacks, and they have the same nutritional qualities of the plain beans; however, they are high in fat and calories. Use them sparingly, in breads and baked goods.

Miso

Miso is a fermented soybean paste that is made by mixing soybeans, salt, water, and a *koji* or cultured grain (usually rice or barley) as a starter. A tablespoon of miso has sixty to eighty calories and virtually no fat; however, it is quite high in sodium and should be used sparingly.

There are several types of miso, which vary in taste and usage depending on the color. Darker shades tend to be stronger and denser than the lighter varieties, which are normally sweeter and less salty. Miso can be used like bouillon to flavor soups; it can be added to sauces for vegetables and to salad dressings; and it can be used to marinate meat for barbecues.

Chinese and Southeast Asian stores sell miso in jars and packages. It will keep for up to a year if stored in an airtight container in the refrigerator.

Tofu

Tofu, or bean curd, as it is sometimes called, is made from soy milk. Dried soybeans are crushed and boiled, and a curdling agent such as nigari or calcium sulfate is added to separate the curds from the whey. The pieces of curd are then poured into square molds, where they become firm.

Tofu is a nutritional powerhouse. It's high in protein (a half cup provides 10 grams), it's rich in essential fats, and it's a good source of zinc, iron, B vitamins, and calcium (if it is made with calcium sulfate). By itself, tofu has no flavor, so it's a natural additive to any healthy, tasty recipe.

Tofu must be kept cool and consumed within two days of opening. A few companies now package tofu in aseptic containers that need no refrigeration and have a shelf life of ten months. See Resources, in the back of the book, for information.

You'll discover several forms of tofu in the refrigerated section of the market:

Silken or *soft tofu* has a creamy consistency and is best for soups, desserts, sauces, and some delicate dishes requiring a smooth texture. Blend it into drinks, puddings, and pureed vegetables.

Firm tofu handles cutting quite well and can be added to vegetable dishes, stews, chili, and casseroles.

Hard tofu can be deep-fried, marinated for barbecuing, and crumbled into salads or into toppings for pasta.

Deep-fried tofu puffs are small cubes of tofu, light brown in color. They are very light and airy inside and can be eaten straight from the package with a soy or chili sauce or added to soups, stews, and stuffings. They can also be cut up into smaller sizes and added to salads, much like croutons in a Caesar salad. Notice that they are deep-fried and thus should be used sparingly.

Tofu desserts, mayonnaise, cream cheese, yogurt, and *dips* are among some of the new products made with tofu. Some of these are wonderful substitutes for the traditional products. Do check the labels for fat content and other added ingredients. Just because it advertises itself as a tofu or soy product does not necessarily mean it is healthy.

Soy Flour

Soy flour is made from the dehulled soybean, which is milled, toasted, and ground. Full-fat soy flour is very high in fat, so look for defatted flour, from which the oil has been extracted during processing. Defatted soy flour is not only lower in calories and fat than ordinary wheat flour, but is also higher in protein.

Soy flour is heavier than wheat flour and is creamy in color; it has a distinctive "beany" smell that usually translates into a rather nutty flavor after cooking. Cakes, biscuits, and cookies can be made from soybean flour, but you'll want to use it in combination with a lighter flour. To see how it works, try substituting about 20 percent of the wheat flour with soy flour in one of your tested favorite recipes (soy flour can substitute for between 30 and 50 percent of the regular flour in your recipes). You may need to add a bit more moisture if the dough seems too dry. Note that since soy flour typically browns more quickly than wheat flour, lowering baking temperature by twenty-five degrees may be necessary. Soy flour does not contain gluten, so you cannot substitute it entirely for wheat flour in yeast breads.

Because soy flour is gluten-free, it's a good alternative for individuals with celiac disease. Store soy flour in the refrigerator or freezer until you are ready to use it.

Soy Protein Powder

This readily available soy product is made from defatted soy flakes, containing about 90 percent protein. It can be added to smoothies or breakfast drinks to boost your intake of plant protein and phytoestrogens (PE). Most powders contain in excess of 2 mg of isoflavones (a subclass of PE) in each gram of soy protein powder. There is a whole range of brands available in health-food stores and by direct mail order (see page 66 for some of the common brands and their isoflavone contents). Soy protein powder is often added to meal-replacement bars, high-protein replacement drink powders, or body-building protein products. Unfortunately, the phytoestrogen content is not always listed on the product.

Soy Sauce

Soy sauce is made from salted, roasted soybeans that have been fermented for a few months or up to a year in huge vats. It is said that the sauce tastes better if the container is made of wood.

There are basically two types of soy sauce, light and dark. Both types are used in Chinese cooking, while in several other nations, light soy is the only type widely used. The lighter soy sauce is normally used for marinating meat, fish, and poultry, and for making sauces. Dark soy sauce, which is thick and viscous from the inclusion of molasses, is reserved for richer stews and sauces. Generally, dark soy sauce is sweeter and less salty, and it gives meat a lustrous, dark-brown color. The manufacturer may add black beans to the processing; this is known as black-bean soy sauce. Mushrooms are sometimes added to the soy sauce extracts during processing, producing mushroom soy sauce. The soy sauce brands most commonly available in North American supermarkets (Kikkoman, La Choy, etc.) are light soy sauces. At Asian groceries in the U.S. you can obtain not only dark soy sauce, but also the more delicate-flavored light soys imported from China, Hong Kong, and Taiwan (brands such as Pearl River, Superior Soy, and Amoy). If there is no Asian market nearby, tamari (a very rich Japanese soy sauce) is available at most health-food stores and makes a passable substitute for dark soy. Add a generous pinch of sugar to any recipe in which you are substituting a light soy or tamari for dark soy.

Soy sauce is low in isoflavones, so it is not considered a potent phytonutrient, like the other soy products. It is high in salt and should be used sparingly, especially if you suffer from high blood pressure or kidney disorders. You can find low-salt versions; check the labels.

Soybean Sprouts

This product must not be confused with mung bean sprouts, which are readily available in most supermarkets. Soybean sprouts, which you can buy in packages from Asian food stores and specialty stores, take longer to cook than mung bean sprouts. Their roots are slightly stringy, and the cotyledons (seed leaves) are very bright yellow in color and thick and broad in structure. This part of the sprout contains the most nutrients and gives it a very nutty taste.

Weight for weight, the phytoestrogen (coumestrol) content in soybean sprouts is at least fourteen times greater than that in alfalfa sprouts and seventy times greater than that in frozen green or string beans. Like the mung bean sprout, the soybean sprout is also a good source of vitamin C.

Both beans can be sprouted at home at your convenience. Should you care to experiment, purchase very fresh soybeans and presoak them in cold water overnight. Sow onto a supporting porous bed in a clean container, and keep in an airy place away from direct sunlight. Water twice daily and drain the water so that the sprouting beans are not water-logged, nor does the sprouting tray ever dry out completely. The bean sprouts will be ready to harvest in four days. Remove the skin before cooking. The sprouts can be kept for two days in the refrigerator after harvesting.

Lecithin

Lecithin is a byproduct of soybean oil. It is a natural emulsifier used in the manufacture of a wide variety of products, such as candy, bakery products, chocolate coatings, and margarine. Lecithin is gaining popularity in the health field because of its antioxidant properties and potential cholesterol-lowering effect.

Lecithin is available in powdered and granular forms and in tablets, often combined with other vitamins and minerals. You can add the powder or granules to milk shakes, eggnogs, soups, and salads, or sprinkle them over your breakfast cereal.

Soybean Oil

Soybean oil is an extract from soybeans. Although soybean oil does not contain isoflavones, it is rich in omega-3 and omega-6 fatty acids, as well as linolenic and linoleic acid, which are said to help prevent bowel and breast cancers. Oil derived from soy has a light, bland flavor and a high smoking point that makes it attractive for stir-frying vegetables, which requires high heat. Many commercial products are made with soybean oil, such as baked goods, prepared foods, and salad dressings.

Tempeh

Tempeh is made from fermented soybeans, usually mixed with a grain such as rice or millet. It has a meatlike texture and tastes nutty, somewhat like a mushroom. Tempeh can be marinated for grilling or barbecuing. Chunks of tempeh can also be added to chili or spaghetti sauce, or pan-fried with mushrooms, onions, and breadcrumbs for a delicious stuffing. It can be grated and made into vegetarian burgers or diced and added to salads.

Tempeh is a rich source of protein, fiber, isoflavones, iron, potassium, calcium, and B vitamins, particularly vitamin B-12, which is usually found only in foods of animal origin.

Soy Grits

Soy grits are made by removing the soybeans' skin prior to lightly steaming and grinding them. They taste much like soybeans and have a similar nutritional value. Because their texture is similar to ground beef, they are a good substitute in meat dishes such as chili, meat loaf, stew, casseroles, and spaghetti sauce.

Texturized Soy or Vegetable Protein

TSP or TVP is compressed soy flour that is used to extend ground beef dishes such as meat loaf, chili, and hamburgers. TSP is an excellent source of soy protein (1 ounce provides 16 grams) and isoflavones. Its real bonus is that it has almost no fat. TSP products have varying levels of plant estrogens, depending on how they were processed. TSP must be rehydrated before using, and it keeps up to four days in the refrigerator once made.

Other Soy Products

Every month seems to bring new and improved soy products to the shelves of the supermarket and the advertisements in health magazines. Soy cheeses are taking up residence alongside regular cheeses. They look like cheese and come in a good selection, from mild to red-pepper hot. Try them as a substitute in your recipes for quiche, pizza, and lasagna, or just eat them as a snack on crackers.

Soy protein can mimic a variety of meat foods, and they can look, feel, and almost taste like the genuine item. Soy-based hot dogs, sausage, and vegetarian hamburgers are creeping into local markets. While these lookalikes are usually lower in fat than the real thing, they are a poor source of isoflavones, and unless fortified they do not have the same nutritional content as the other, purer soy products.

Check out some of the other varieties of soy: soy mayonnaise, cookies, breads, crackers, yogurt, and smoothies.

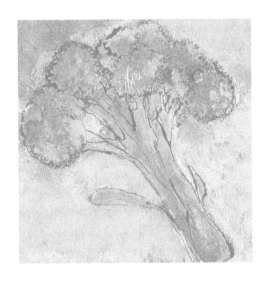

Chapter Four

Integrating *Natural* Estrogens into Your Life

T here are no official guidelines regarding natural estrogen intake in the daily diet, no recommended daily allowances or space allotted on the food pyramid. Official guidelines may be drawn up in the future as new scientific information becomes available and new standards are accepted. However, it may take another generation of scientists' work to steer us accurately through such a complicated maze. The following general recommendations are based on current knowledge derived from decades of research by various dedicated food scientists:

◈ For general good health, consume at least one or two servings of soy per day, aiming for a total of 30 to 50 milligrams of isoflavones. On average, each gram of soy protein may contain 1 to 3 milligrams of phytoestrogens. Recall from earlier chapters that the genetic origin of the soy plants, their season of harvest, and the climatic and environmental conditions under which they were grown all influence phytoestrogen concentration.

Those who worry about fat content can look for fat-reduced varieties of soy foods. In general, defatting of soy products does not significantly affect their phytoestrogen content.

Here are a few suggestions for serving sizes:

½ cup tofu or tempeh
3½ tablespoons soy protein powder
1 cup soy milk
½ cup cooked dried soybeans
½ cup dry-roasted soy nuts
¼ cup TVP (reconstituted)
1 soy burger
2 soy hot dogs

◈ Consuming excessive amounts of natural-estrogen foods, such as four to five times the average Asian daily intake, is not necessarily more beneficial, as improvements in serum cholesterol, blood pressure, hot flashes, and other menopausal symptoms do not bear a linear relationship to one's intake. Flooding all of your estrogen receptor sites with excessive phytoestrogens may actually produce an antiestrogenic response. So, eat in moderation.

◈ Make it a practice to eat different foods each day. A variety of foods are known to contain phytoestrogens, and those not yet tested may also contain these beneficial substances. Although grains, spices, fruits, and vegetables possess smaller amounts of phytoestrogens than soy, this does not mean they are ineffective, especially if many of these foods are ingested in the same day. In Asian diets, rice, barley, and other grains, seeds, beans, legumes, sprouts, tea, and seafood are featured in every meal. Vary your grains, fruits, and vegetables to get the most out of plant estrogens.

◈ Moderation with any food is best. Overindulgence in one particular foodstuff to the exclusion of other food groups can produce side effects. For example, an individual who eats excessive amounts of carrots, pumpkin, or corn can manifest carotenemia and turn orange; more importantly, in a young menstruating female, this condition can cause the cessation of periods (amenorrhea). Once the excess intake has stopped for a few months, normal function will resume.

◈ Broad-spectrum antibiotics kill friendly bacteria in the bowel; therefore, if you're taking antibiotics, plant estrogens may be unavailable for absorption even though you've eaten adequate quantities of estrogen-rich foods. It may take two to six weeks for your system to recover after a course of antibiotics. Do not panic when hot flashes and menopausal symptoms reappear after a bout of antibiotics; it is only a temporary setback.

◈ Women experiencing sore breasts on the natural estrogen diet should avoid foods and beverages containing caffeine, as these tend to aggravate breast tenderness and lumpiness. If your periods are heavy, avoid foods containing high amounts of salicylates, such as tomatoes, oranges, and pineapples. Salicylates thin the blood and aggravate heavy menstrual flow. Resume your usual diet after a break of four to five days.

⟜ General Health Guidelines ⟞

Some of the following information is repetitive; that's intentional. The basic pearls of wisdom bear repeating because we all have a penchant for forgetting the obvious.

The natural estrogen diet is primarily plant-based. Whether you choose to go vegetarian is up to you. Here are a few guidelines for establishing your own personal plan.

- *Whole grains*: seven to ten servings/day (one serving = one-half cup grain, cereal, or pasta, or one slice bread)

- *Legumes*: seven or more servings/week (one serving = one-half cup cooked beans)

- *Fruits*: two to three servings/day (one serving = one piece of fresh fruit, one-half cup cooked fruit, or three-quarters cup fruit juice)

- *Vegetables*: three to four servings/day (one serving = one-half cup cooked or one cup raw vegetables)

- *Soy foods*: one to two servings/day (one serving = one cup soy milk, one-half cup tofu, tempeh, or green beans)

- *Meat, chicken, and fish*: no more than six ounces/day

- *Fiber*: A high-fiber diet helps to prevent breast cancer and maintain a healthy heart. Total intake per day should range between 25 and 40 grams. The chart below shows the amount of fiber found in common foods.

Fiber Content of Some Common Foods

Cereal
½ cup high-fiber cereal = 14 grams
½ cup medium-fiber cereal = 8 grams

Beans
¾ cup of most beans = 14 grams
10 ounces split-pea soup = 4 grams

Fiber Content of Some Common Foods (cont'd.)

Breads

1 slice whole-wheat bread = 2 grams

Fruit

1 medium apple = 4 grams
8 dried apricots = 3 grams
1 large banana = 2 grams

Vegetables

1 large baked potato = 4 grams
½ cup cooked broccoli = 2 grams

❖ Keep total fats in your diet between 20 and 30 percent of total calories per day. If you are eating approximately two thousand calories per day, this translates to 44 to 66 grams of fat each day. Minimize saturated, trans, and polyunsaturated fats, and emphasize monounsaturated fats and fish oils or omega 3-fatty acids.

❖ Exercise is a must. Do it for your heart, breasts, mind, and soul. Exercise helps to control estrogen activity in the body, decreasing harmful estrogen and increasing healthy estrogen. Shoot for about five hours a week of some activity that you enjoy. Vary your exercise just as you vary your foods. To work different muscles, mix an aerobic-type, heartbeat-raising activity with something that stresses and strengthens the muscles.

❖ Calcium and magnesium help to build the bones and possibly lower blood pressure. Premenopausal women need 1,000 milligrams daily, and menopausal women require 1,500 milligrams. Your magnesium intake should be 500 to 650 milligrams per day (about half the dose of calcium). Take the two together in a combined supplement, and divide your doses into morning and nighttime supplements.

- Excessive salt, sugar, alcohol, caffeine, and soda pop have been reported to negatively affect bone density. Excessive alcohol (more than two glasses a day) is associated with an increased risk of breast cancer and osteoporosis. Minimize these in your diet.

- Drink about eight glasses of water each day. Water delivers nutrients to the cells, enables your glands and hormones to operate more efficiently, allows your liver to break down fat, releases excess water by causing you to urinate more, and keeps your skin and organs hydrated. Don't wait for nature to signal thirst; sip throughout the day.

- Get adequate sleep and rest. You will feel and look better. Our bodies and minds need time to repair and regenerate them-selves. Avoid sedatives and pills, which artificially induce sleep. A warm glass of soy milk is helpful before bed, rather than a cup of coffee or tea (unless it's herb tea). The caffeine in tea and coffee tends to stimulate some people, making them restless and causing difficulties in falling asleep.

- Don't smoke. If you do, make a commitment to quit. Smoking increases the incidence of heart disease, hypertension, osteo-porosis, lung cancer, and possibly breast cancer.

- Schedule regular checkups with your doctor. Have your choles-terol levels tested, making sure you get the full panel and not just the total cholesterol count. If you haven't already done it, go in for a bone-density baseline test so that you and your doc-tor can monitor your bone health. If you are older than forty, have a mammography screening at least every two years; some special situations call for yearly checks. And, of course, don't forget your annual Pap smear.

- Perform monthly breast self-examinations. The best time is fol-lowing your period (if you are still having menstrual periods). If you don't have periods or if you've had a hysterectomy, pick a particular day of the month, such as the first or the last, and check yourself regularly on that day. If you find a lump, do not panic; make an appointment with your doctor to have it checked. Take along any old X rays of the breast that you may have, or retrieve them from labs where they may be stored. The doctor and radiologist need to compare these to the new ones they'll take to determine if there have been any changes.

❧ Develop a positive attitude toward menopause and aging. Menopause is a natural phase of a woman's life. Some cultures look upon menopausal women with great respect and regard them as sources of wisdom. It is a time free from the fear of pregnancy and free from the chores of childbearing and child rearing (for most women). It is new territory filled with different experiences and lessons. Prepare for it as much as you can, and learn to enjoy all that life has to offer.

⤙ Not for Women Only ⤚

Although the natural estrogen diet is primarily aimed at perimenopausal and menopausal women, its health benefits extend to men, children, and other women. In men, added benefits include a decreased risk of prostate and bowel cancer. In premenopausal women, benefits include minimizing premenstrual symptoms and lowering the risk of breast and bowel cancer. In general, one or two servings of soy foods a day for men, children, and premenopausal women is adequate for cardiac and blood pressure benefits.

⤙ Soy the Quick and Easy Way ⤚

Sometimes it's just hard to get a new program going. We are so driven by habit that trying new foods may be difficult, and the mere thought of altering our comfortable routines may seem even more unappealing. This book helps you ease into the natural estrogen diet by offering suggestions that you can start tomorrow, without altering your usual routines too dramatically. After you've made small changes and gained courage, you can move on to some of the suggestions that you'd bypassed, or you might even experiment with some of the wonderful recipes found later in the book. The book also provides nutritional information for specific soy products, so you will be aware of the caloric, fat, fiber, and calcium content of these foods.

Below are some recommendations for integrating natural estrogen foods into each of your daily meals.

Snacks

- Soy nuts
- Soy milk, flavored or plain
- Fresh green soybeans, or *edamame*
- Soy yogurt
- Soy cheese on pita bread, tortillas, or crackers
- Smoothies made with soy protein powder or pureed tofu and your favorite fruits
- Trail mix (oats, rice, wheat, sunflower seeds, nuts)
- Carrots and cucumbers
- Apples, pears, grapes, and plums
- Papayas
- Muffins or pancakes made with soy flour (substitute soy flour for 20 percent of total flour)

Breakfast

- Crumble firm tofu in skillet and cook like scrambled eggs.
- Pour soy milk on high-fiber cereal.
- Mix soy yogurt into high-fiber cereal.
- Sprinkle flaxseed on high-fiber cereal.
- Sprinkle isolated soy protein (ISP) on cereal or fruit.
- Add ISP to baked goods.
- Blend two to four tablespoons of ISP into orange juice.
- Add prunes to high-fiber cereal, or eat plain.

Lunch/Dinner

- Add fresh green soybeans to salads.
- Substitute soy milk for white sauce or pudding, or use as a base for cream soup.
- Use blended tofu as a base for cream soup.
- Cube firm tofu and add to soups, stews, casseroles, or chili.
- Eat takeout miso soup, or make it yourself (see the recipe on page 106).
- Substitute creamed tofu for cheese in lasagna or enchiladas.
- Marinate firm tofu and grill, or make into kebobs.
- Grill tempeh like a burger.
- Add tofu or tempeh to vegetable soup.
- Stir-fry firm tofu with vegetables.
- Eat lentil or split-pea soup.
- Add carrots, beets, or cucumbers to salads.
- Spoon tofu chili over a baked potato.
- Make chili dogs from soy hot dogs and vegetarian chili; top with soy cheese.
- Add soy hot dogs to bean or pea soups.
- Make tofu tacos with crumbled firm tofu and taco spices.
- Buy or make soy burgers; serve on wheat bun with lettuce, tomatoes, and onion.
- Make or buy low-fat coleslaw.

Nutritional Content of Soy Foods

	Soy protein (grams)	Fat (grams)	Calories
miso (1 tablespoon)	2	1	35
soy flour (3½ ounces)			
regular	35	22	441
defatted	47	1.2	329
soy milk (1 cup)			
regular	10	4	140
reduced fat	4	2	100
soy nuts (1 ounce)	13.3	5.5	127
soybean oil (1 tablespoon)	0	13.6	120
soy sprouts (½ cup)	4.6	2.5	45
soybeans, dried	14.3	7.7	149
(½ cup, cooked)			
soybeans, green, without pods	6	2	60
(½ cup, cooked)			
tofu (½ cup)			
firm	13	6	120
soft	9	5	80
silken	9.6	2.4	72
tempeh (½ cup)	17	8	204
TVP (1 cup, reconstituted)	22	0.2	120

Nutritional Content of Brand-Name Soy Drinks and Foods

Drinks (1 cup unless indicated; each cup has approximately 300 milligrams of calcium)	*Soy protein (grams)*	*Fat (grams)*	*Calories*
Edensoy Extra Original Soy Milk	10	4	130
Pacific Lite Plain	4	2.5	100
Pacific Lite Cocoa	4	2	160
Revival Soy Meal-Replacement Drink	20	2.5	240
Solair Vanilla Bean	3	2	98
Trader Joe's Soy-Um	4	3	100
VitaSoy Enriched Original	6	3	110
VitaSoy Enriched Vanilla	6	3	140
West Soy Dessert Drink (6 fl. ounces)	6	4	160

Foods			
Boca Burger (original; 1)	12	0	84
Fantastic Foods Mandarin Chow Mein with Tofu (1 package)	22	5	330
Hickory Baked Tofu (3 ounces)	18	3.5	140
Light Life Smart Dogs (1)	9	0	45
Morningstar Breakfast Links (2)	n/a	5	90
Nancy's Soy Yogurt (8 ounces)	7	4	200
Trader Joe's Eggless Salad (1/2 cup)	7	8	120
TofuRella Tofu Cheese (1 ounce)	6	5	80
Wildwood Tofu Cutlets (3 ounces)	13	12	180
Wildwood Veggie Burger (1)	11	10	150
Yamato Boiled Soybeans (1/2 cup)	9	5	103
Yves Veggie Cuisine Tofu Wieners (1)	9	0	45

Nutritional Content of Brand-Name Soy Drinks and Foods

Soy powders	Soy protein (grams)	Isoflavones (milligrams)
Genisoy Natural Protein Powder (1 ounce)	24	74
Genisoy Soy Protein Shake (1 ounce)	14	43
Health Source Soy Protein Shake, Vanilla (1 ounce)	20	55
Twinlab Isoflavone Powder (1 teaspoon)	34	85
Whole Foods Soy Protein Powder (1 ounce)	24	43

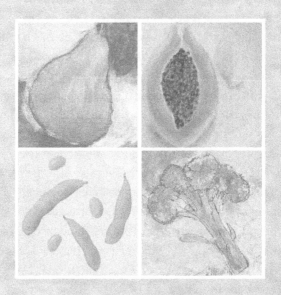

Part Two

Recipes

T elling someone to eat more soy is good advice. But showing you how to actually do it is another matter. In this part of the book, we have compiled delicious, practical, and easy-to-prepare dishes incorporating soy products and other phytoestrogen-rich foods. Choose the recipes you think you'll like, based on the ingredients you already know, and then experiment with something new and exotic. After gaining confidence in phytoestrogen cooking, venture out and create your own dishes with the various soy products that are available in supermarkets. We hope you will be encouraged and inspired by your new cooking experiences.

The nutrient analysis for the original recipes in the Australian edition was calculated by Jenny Chan, a practicing consultant dietitian and nutritionist in Liverpool, New South Wales, Australia. Additional recipes from various contributors were arranged and annotated by Naomi Wise. The nutritional analyses of all of the recipes in the first U.S. edition were calculated by Amy Demmon using the Nutritional Data Resources Nutrient Data Base. In this second U.S. edition, the nutrition analyses of all recipes new to this edition and all recipes that have been modified since the publication of the first U.S. edition were calculated by Linda Yoakam, M.S., R.D., L.D., using Nutritionist Pro software. These analyses do not include optional variations. Equivalents for certain ingredients in the first U.S. edition were supplied by Linda Ojeda.

People watching their weight can use low-fat soy milk and defatted soy flour in these recipes, although the latter can be difficult to find. Hopefully, defatted soy flour will become a common item in supermarkets and food stores in the future.

Those of you cooking for several people in a household can add chicken or other meat to the recipes so that the rest of your family won't miss out on their preferred protein. For example, in stir-fry dishes using tempeh or tofu cutlet, add some diced chicken for those who may prefer it. Lastly, those who are allergic to or intolerant of certain ingredients in the recipes should substitute or omit the offending ingredient from the recipe.

Always try to consume whole, organic foods; the less processed a food is and the fewer chemicals and pesticides it contains, the better. Food processing can result in the addition of unwanted chemicals that the body must deal with, transforming healthy foods to unhealthy ones. Make sure your chicken, meat, and eggs are hormone-free. When selecting tofu, choose the ones made with either calcium sulfate or nigari. Use naturally brewed soy sauce even though it is more expensive than the non-brewed variety.

⋙ Phytoestrogen Content ⋘

The phytoestrogen (PE) content of each recipe is listed in a table beginning on page 71. The PE content was calculated using the USDA–Iowa State University isoflavones database, and also from W. Mazur's report on phytoestrogen content in foods, which includes lignans as well as isoflavones. Data from the USDA were obtained from various scientific papers, and an average phytoestrogen value was computed after converting the glycoside forms to the aglycone forms. Since the weights of specific food items in Mazur's paper were presented as dry weights, we converted the values to wet weights, using the usual moisture content of the foods.

It should be noted that the three classes of phytoestrogens—isoflavones, lignans, and coumestrol—all have different estrogen potencies. (See page 224 for a diagram illustrating how some of the different phytoestrogens are grouped.) When tested in a lab with cell cultures, for example, coumestrol is 15½ times more potent than daidzein, genistein 6½ times more potent, and equol 4½ times. We are unsure whether the relative potencies remain exactly the same after ingestion. At the current stage of research, it remains impossible to figure out a common phytoestrogen denominator. Therefore, the PE content given in the recipes contains the sum total of the three PEs (isoflavones, lignans, and coumestrol). Furthermore, it is impossible to be exact when estimating the PE content of each foodstuff, as the PE content varies based on individual batches, season of growth, time of harvest, amount of processing, storage time, fermentation, and other factors, as discussed in Part I of the book. The amounts we've included in this book can be considered fairly reliable estimates.

The PE content of each recipe is rated using stars, as follows:

PE content	PE star rating
0–5 mg	★
5–10 mg	★★
10–15 mg	★★★
15–20 mg	★★★★
20–25 mg	★★★★★
Over 25 mg	★★★★★+

(The star ratings appear on each page next to the recipes.)

In order to achieve between 40 and 50 milligrams of PE per day, then, one should aim for enough servings of food to add up to a total of ten stars. Since the PE content per gram of soy protein varies between 1 and 3 milligrams, this grading system does not precisely reflect the amount of soy protein contained in the recipe. However, as a general rule, 25 grams of soy protein may translate to between 25 and 75 milligrams of PE.

Note in the following table that for a few recipes, the quantity on which the PE content is based differs from the individual serving size noted in the recipe itself. For example, whereas the recipe for Chickpea Dip (Hummus) yields about 10 servings of 3 tablespoons each (and the nutritional information that accompanies the recipe is based on the serving size of 3 tablespoons), the PE content rating is based on 1 cup of the dip.

In other cases, where the number of servings can vary for a recipe, the PE ratings for both portion sizes are given. For example, the creamy potato soup can serve four or six, depending on the serving size. If the whole recipe is divided into four servings, the PE rating for a single serving is three (★★★); if the whole recipe is divided into six servings, the PE rating per serving is two (★★). This is because the total PE content for the recipe is 55.3 milligrams. Divide this by 4, and you get 13.8 milligrams per serving; divide it by 6, and you get 9.2 milligrams per serving.

Phytoestrogen Content of Recipes

Recipe	Page No.	Recipe yield, or number of servings	PE rating	Quantity on which PE rating is based
Chickpea Dip (Hummus)	94	1⅔ cups	★	Per cup
Soybean Dip	95	¾ cup or 6 servings	★★★★★+ ★★★	Per ¼ cup Per serving
Spicy Lentil Dip	96	1½ cups	★	Per cup
Spring Rolls	97	10 servings	★	Per recipe
Grilled Soy Cheese Sandwiches	99	1 sandwich	★★★	Per serving
Soy-Banana Breakfast Drink	100	1 serving of about 1½ cups each	★★★★	Per cup
Cantaloupe–Soy Milk Shake	101	2 servings of about 1½ cups each	★★★★★+ ★★★★★	Per serving Per cup
Strawberry Soy Drink	102	1 serving of about 1¾ cups each	★★★★★	Per cup
Tropical Fruit Smoothie	103	2 servings of about 1½ cups each	★★★★	Per cup
Miso Soup	106	1 serving	★★★★★+	Per serving
Creamy Corn Soup	107	6 servings	★★	Per serving
Tomato Corn Chowder	108	6 servings	★★	Per serving
Creamy Tomato Soup	109	3 servings	★★★★★+	Per serving

Recipe	Page No.	Recipe yield, or number of servings	PE rating	Quantity on which PE rating is based
Creamy Pumpkin Soup	110	6 servings	★★	Per serving
Lentil-Vegetable Soup	111	6 servings	★	Per serving
Creamy Potato Soup	112	6 servings	★★	Per serving
Curried Carrot Soup	113	4 servings	★	Per serving
Tofu and Watercress Soup	114	4 servings	★★★★★	Per serving
Healthy Potato Leek Soup	115	6 servings	★★	Per serving
Seafood Tofu Soup	116	4 servings	★★★★★	Per serving
Split Pea and Carrot Soup	117	4 servings	★	Per serving
Chickpea Salad	121	6 servings	★	Per serving
Bean Salad	122	6 servings	★★★★	Per serving
Thai Salad	123	4 servings	★★★	Per serving
Apple and Potato Salad	124	8 servings	★	Per serving
Soy Macaroni Salad	125	6 servings	★★	Per serving
Greek Tofu Salad	126	4 servings	★★★★	Per serving
Green Soybean Salad	127	4 servings	★★★	Per serving
Summertime Pickled Curried Vegetables	128	12 servings	★	Per serving
Cabbage Rolls	130	6 rolls	★★★	Per roll
Tofu Mayonnaise	131	12 tbs.	★★★★★+	Per ½ cup

Recipe	Page No.	Recipe yield, or number of servings	PE rating	Quantity on which PE rating is based
Creamy Poppy Seed Dressing	132	2½ cups	★★	Per ½ cup
Healthy Caesar Salad Dressing	133	1 cup	★★★★	Per ½ cup
Creamy Basil Dressing	134	2 cups	★★★	Per ½ cup
Curried Chickpeas	135	6 servings	★	Per serving
Spicy Chickpeas	137	4 servings to 6 servings	★★	Per serving
Soy Samosas	138	24 samosas	★★	Per 3 samosas
Stir-Fried Green Beans with Pine Nuts	139	4 servings	★	Per serving
Asian Tofu Salad	140	4 servings	★★★	Per serving
Five Spiced Tofu	141	4 servings	★★★★	Per serving
Bean Sprouts in Fish Sauce	142	4 servings	★	Per serving
Cheesy Scalloped Potatoes	143	8 servings	★	Per serving
Tofu in Pastry Baskets	144	4 servings	★★	Per serving
Fried Rice	146	6 servings	★	Per serving
Gado Gado	149	8 servings	★★★	Per serving
Hot Pot (Steamboat)	151	8 servings	★★★★★	Per serving
Poached Spiced Chicken	155	4 servings	★	Per serving
Spiced Roast Chicken	157	2 servings	★	Per serving

Recipe	Page No.	Recipe yield, or number of servings	PE rating	Quantity on which PE rating is based
Teriyaki Chicken	158	4 servings	★	Per serving
Sesame Chicken	159	4 servings	★	Per serving
Chicken Breasts with Chipotle Sauce	160	4 servings	★★★	Per serving
Tacos	162	6 servings	★★★★	Per serving
Festive Vegetable Fajita Wraps	163	4 servings	★★★★★+	Per serving
Healthy Chili	164	8 servings	★★★	Per serving
Curried Tofu and Vegetables	165	6 servings	★★	Per serving
Vegetable Tofu Stir-Fry	166	4 servings	★★★★★	Per serving
Tofu in Oyster Sauce	167	4 servings	★★★★★	Per serving
Tofu with Ground Meat	168	4 servings	★★★★★	Per serving
Hunanese Tofu Beef	170	4 servings	★★★★★+	Per serving
Steamed Fish with Tofu	171	4 servings	★★★★★	Per serving
Sweet and Sour Tofu	172	4 servings	★★★★★	Per serving
Tofu and Mushroom Parcels	173	4 servings	★★★★	Per serving
Stir-Fried Baby Bok Choy and Tofu	174	2 servings	★★★★	Per serving
Eight-Treasured Chap Choy	175	4 servings	★★	Per serving
Eggplant in Miso Sauce	176	3 servings	★★★★	Per serving
Baked Fish in Miso Sauce	177	2 servings	★★	Per serving

Recipe	Page No.	Recipe yield, or number of servings	PE rating	Quantity on which PE rating is based
Corn Bread Tamale Pie	178	4 servings to 6 servings	★★★★★+ ★★★★	Per serving
Stewed Bean Curd Skin and Cloud Ears with Pork	180	6 servings	★★★★★+	Per serving
Stir-Fried Tempeh and Vegetables	182	2 servings	★★★★★	Per serving
Stir-Fried Prawns, Snow Peas, and Tofu	183	4 servings	★★★★	Per serving
Tofu Cutlet in Lettuce Leaves with Prawns	184	6 servings	★★	Per serving
Soybean Sprouts with Ground Meat	185	4 servings	★★★★★+	Per serving
Soybean Sprouts with Shredded Beef	187	4 servings	★★★★★+	Per serving
Soybean Sprouts with Shrimp	188	4 servings	★★★★★+	Per serving
Baked Soybeans in Eggplant	189	2 servings	★★★★★	Per serving
Stir-Fried Rice Noodles with Tofu Cutlet	190	4 servings	★★	Per serving
Stir-Fried Chinese Cabbage and Bean Thread Noodles	191	6 servings	★	Per serving
Mediterranean Spinach Pasta	193	4 servings	★★★★★+	Per serving
Sesame Tofu and Spinach Pasta	194	3 servings	★★★★	Per serving
Easy Vegetable Lasagna	195	8 servings to 10 servings	★★ ★	Per serving

Recipe	Page No.	Recipe yield, or number of servings	PE rating	Quantity on which PE rating is based
Tuna Soy-Mac Casserole	196	with soy cheese: 4 servings / with Cheddar cheese: 4 servings	★★★★★+ / ★★★★★	Per serving
Soy Pancakes	198	6 servings	★★★★	Per serving
Banana Oat Pancakes	199	6 servings (2 pancakes each)	★★★	Per serving
Crusty Soy Bread	200	14 slices	★ / ★★★★	Per slice / Per quarter loaf
Herb and Cheese Focaccia	201	6 servings	★★	Per serving
Cherry Muffins	202	10 muffins to 12 muffins	★★ / ★★	Per muffin
Apple Muffins	203	10 muffins to 12 muffins	★★ / ★★	Per muffin
Banana Oatmeal Muffins	204	12 muffins	★★	Per muffin
Sweet Potato Muffins	205	12 muffins	★	Per muffin
Little Lemon and Green Tea Muffins	206	24 small muffins	★	Per muffin
Double Chocolate Muffins	207	12 muffins	★★★	Per muffin
Fruity Soy Scones	208	4 servings	★★★	Per serving (2 scones)

Recipe	Page No.	Recipe yield, or number of servings	PE rating	Quantity on which PE rating is based
Soy and Date Scones	209	6 servings	★★★★	Per serving (2 scones)
Strawberry Soy Dessert	212	2 servings	★★★	Per serving
Banana Berry Whip	213	2 servings to 3 servings	★★★★★ ★★★★	Per serving
Baked Honey Custard	214	4 servings to 6 servings	★★★ ★★	Per serving
Soy and Oatmeal Cookies	215	28 cookies	★ ★★	Per cookie Per 3 cookies
Banana-Topped Chocolate Silk Pie	216	10 servings	★★★	Per serving
Heart-Healthy Pumpkin Pie	217	8 servings	★★	Per serving
Soy Apple Cake	218	8 servings	★★★	Per serving
Soy Carrot Cake	219	8 servings	★★	Per serving
Soy Tea Cake	220	6 servings	★★	Per serving
Soy Bread and Butter Pudding	221	4 servings	★★★★★	Per serving
Rich Cocoa Brownies	222	16 brownies	★	Per brownie

Conversion Table

1 teaspoon = 5 milliliters

1 tablespoon = 3 teaspoons = 15 milliliters

1 cup = 8 fluid ounces = 250 milliliters

1 ounce = 30 grams

1 gram = 0.035 ounce

1 inch = 2.5 centimeters

1 centimeter = 0.4 inch

1 fluid ounce = 30 milliliters

20 fluid ounces = 2 ½ cups = 625 milliliters

Abbreviations:	g: grams	mL: milliliter	mm: millimeter
kg: kilogram	L: liter	cm: centimeter	

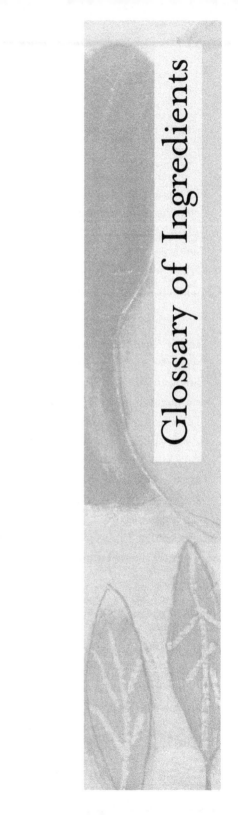

Glossary of Ingredients

❧ CHICKPEAS (GARBANZO BEANS) ❧

Chickpeas come cooked, in cans, or dried, in packages. They are very rich in phytoestrogens, protein, and fiber. To cook dried chickpeas, see page 86.

❧ CHILI SAUCE ❧

Chinese chili sauce is not the same as America's mild, tomatoey bottled chili sauce (for shrimp cocktails, etc.); nor is it a puree like some bottled Asian hot sauces. In Asian groceries and supermarkets with Asian food sections, look for bottled dark-red sauce in which large quantities of chopped red hot peppers are visible. Vietnamese chili sauce is similar to Chinese. See page 153 for a homemade version.

❧ COOKING OILS ❧

In the Asian recipes in this book, and for recipes requiring deep-frying, we have indicated a choice of soybean oil, peanut oil, or canola oil. Soybean oil contains phytoestrogens, but it is polyunsaturated (not recommended for health reasons). Moreover, it is not always easy to find. Peanut oil is also unsaturated, but it offers the most authentic flavor for Asian dishes. If you are shopping for other ingredients at an Asian grocery, you can find Chinese peanut oils as well; the brand with the richest flavor is Lion and Globe. Canola oil is monounsaturated and the healthiest choice, but it has no flavor of its own to contribute to foods; many people object to a "greasy" aftertaste. Olive oil, which is monounsaturated, has been specified wherever its distinctive flavor would make a positive contribution.

❧ DASHI ❧

Dashi is a Japanese soup bouillon with dried Bonito (fish) powder and powdered seaweeds as the main ingredients. It may also contain other ingredients such as powdered soy sauce, salt, hydrolyzed soybean protein, and glucose. You can get sachets or packets of dashi to use as soup stock. Dashi may also be incorporated into some miso paste (for example, Marukome brand of miso paste) so there is no need to add extra dashi when using this brand of paste to make miso soup.

GARAM MASALA (INDIAN SPICE MIXTURE)

Garam masala is an aromatic Indian spice mixture that's much more widely used in India than curry powder. It's available from Indian food stores, some gourmet shops, and most spice catalogs. To make your own, see page 89.

KETJAP MANIS

Ketjap manis is a sweet, thick soy sauce made in Indonesia. Its name is the basis of the English word *ketchup*. It is available in Asian food stores, specialty food stores, and by mail order from specialty food catalogs.

LOW-FAT GROUND PORK

Store-bought minced pork usually has a very high fat content (up to 30 percent). To decrease the fat content of the meat to that of skinless chicken breast, for each portion of 3½ ounces, substitute 1 center-cut loin pork chop (about 4 ounces boneless or 5 ounces with bone). Remove visible fat, wash meat surface briefly under hot running water (this will remove bacteria), and, if you don't have a meat grinder, whir in a food processor or chop very fine with a knife. For a richer flavor (with somewhat higher fat), use a pork butt steak, trimming visible fat before processing, and picking over food-processed meat to remove any visible strings of unchopped gristle. (With small quantities as are used in this book, it should take just a minute.)

MISO

There are five types of miso paste; the darker the color, the stronger and tangier the flavor. Some brands, such as Marukome, have dashi concentrate included (see description of dashi on the previous page), so there is no need to add dashi when you use them in soup. Please read the contents of the package carefully before making your purchase. Miso is also a tasty ingredient in salad dressings and in sauces for fish; for these purposes, choose miso without added dashi. Miso may be found in health-food stores and Asian food stores, either on the shelves or in the refrigerated section. After opening, store in the refrigerator.

❧ OILS — SEE COOKING OILS ❧

❧ OYSTER SAUCE ❧

Oyster sauce is readily available from most supermarkets and Asian food stores. The sauce is made from extracts of oyster, caramel, and other additives. Brands do vary in content: Some contain MSG and preservatives, while others are preservative-free. Check the label before making your purchase. Once open, store in the refrigerator; or, if the brand has preservatives and you expect to use the bottle quickly, you can store it in a cool cupboard.

❧ PORK, GROUND — SEE LOW-FAT GROUND PORK ❧

❧ SOY SAUCE, LIGHT AND DARK ❧

There are basically two types of Chinese soy sauce, light and dark. Other Asian countries mainly use light soy. The soy sauce brands most commonly available in North American supermarkets (Kikkoman, La Choy, etc.) are light soy sauces. At Asian groceries in the U.S. you can not only obtain dark soy, which is thick and glutinous because of its molasses content, but you can also find the more delicate-flavored light soys imported from China, Hong Kong, and Taiwan (brands such as Pearl River, Superior Soy, and Amoy). If there is no Asian market nearby, tamari (a very rich Japanese soy sauce) is available at most health-food stores and makes a passable substitute for dark soy. Add a generous pinch of sugar or a teaspoon of molasses to any recipe in which you are substituting a light soy or tamari in place of dark soy.

❧ TAHINI ❧

A beige-colored, bottled sauce made from ground or milled sesame seeds, tahini is available from health-food stores, Middle Eastern–style groceries and delis, and many supermarkets. It is very rich in proteins, calcium, phosphorus, and vitamin E. Tahini also contains phytoestrogens. The oil in the tahini tends to separate from the solids, so stir thoroughly before using. Once opened, tahini should be refrigerated to prevent rancidity. Let it return to room temperature before use, as it is very hard to stir when cold.

❧ TAMARIND ❧

Tamarind is a tropical fruit with a tangy flavor. It is used in Asian and Latin-American cuisines. In Asian and Latin-American groceries it's usually sold as a packaged dried fruit or a dried concentrate. Rehydrate it in water, and use as directed in cooking. East Indian food stores sell small bottles of thick liquid tamarind concentrate. The concentrate is convenient to use, but must be refrigerated after opening because in hot weather it may bubble over onto the cupboard shelf, even if the bottle is tightly capped.

❧ TOFU BUK (DEEP-FRIED TOFU) ❧

Ready-fried tofu is sold in packages at Asian food stores. (If you cannot find it ready-made, see recipe, page 90.) Fried tofu is light brown in color and rather spongy in texture.

❧ TOFU CUTLETS ❧

Tofu cutlets are compressed hard tofu that has been marinated in soy sauce or curry sauce and cooked again before packaging. You can often find tofu cutlets next to other tofu products in the refrigerated section of supermarkets or health-food stores. If unavailable, see recipe, page 92.

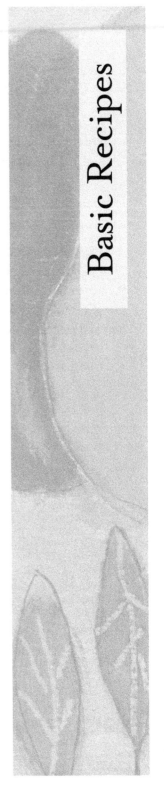

Basic Recipes

Cooked Dried Chickpeas

Note: Cooked chickpeas are used in several recipes in this book. Nutritional information is given in those recipes.

2 cups dried chickpeas (garbanzo beans)
Water, to cover

Place chickpeas in medium saucepan; cover with 2 inches water. Heat to boiling; reduce heat and simmer, uncovered, 2 minutes. Remove from heat and let stand, covered, 1 hour. Drain; return to saucepan and cover with 2 inches cold water. Heat to boiling; reduce heat and simmer, covered, until tender, about 1 hour. Drain.

Cooked chickpeas can be refrigerated for several days before use. Yield: 5–6 cups

COOKED DRIED SOYBEANS

Note: Cooked soybeans are used in several recipes in this book. Nutritional information is given in those recipes.

1 cup dried soybeans
3 ¼ cups water

Soak soybeans overnight in cold water to cover; drain. Rinse and discard any bad beans or debris. Place beans and 3 ¼ cups water in pressure cooker. Heat over high heat until pressurized; reduce heat to low and cook 30 minutes. Release pressure; remove lid and drain. (To cook in saucepan, cover soybeans with 2 inches of water. Heat to boiling; reduce heat and simmer, covered, 2–3 hours, or until tender, adding more water if liquid cooks away.)

Cooked soybeans may be refrigerated or frozen if desired.

Makes about 3 cups.

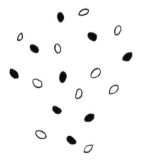

Asian-Style Chicken Stock

PER CUP: 38 CALORIES, 4.8 G PROTEIN, 1.0 G CARBOHYDRATE, 1.4 G FAT (0.4 G SATURATED), 72.0 MG SODIUM, 0.0 G FIBER.

2 pounds bony chicken parts (backs, wing-tips, necks, feet if available)
2½ quarts water
2 slices gingerroot
5 white peppercorns

Place all ingredients in a large saucepan. Heat to boiling; skim gray foam from the top. Reduce heat and simmer, covered, 2–3 hours, or until stock is richly flavored.

Strain stock through fine strainer. Cool; refrigerate covered up to 4 days. Before using, remove fat from surface and discard.

Yield: about 1½ quarts.

Notes: To make stock in a pressure cooker, place ingredients in pressure cooker. Heat over high heat until pressurized; reduce heat and cook 30 minutes. Release pressure; remove lid and strain.

Stock may be frozen for use at a later date. It is convenient to divide it into portions suitable for use in recipes, and only defrost the amount you need. Stock may be frozen in an ice cube tray or in half-cup-sized custard cups. When the stock is frozen, transfer cubes or rounds into freezer bags. Frozen stock keeps for 6 months.

Stock made from bony parts tends to have a higher calcium content. This can be increased by adding 1 tablespoon apple cider vinegar to the cooking pot.

To make beef or pork stock, use 2 pounds meaty beef or pork bones (shanks, shins) instead of chicken; simmer 4–6 hours.

Any fat that you have not skimmed off is very easy to remove once the stock has been chilled.

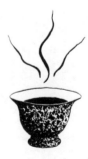

GARAM MASALA

PER TABLESPOON: 20 CALORIES, 0.8 G PROTEIN, 3.5 G CARBOHYDRATE, 0.8 G FAT
(0.0 G SATURATED), 1.9 MG SODIUM, 1.0 G FIBER.

¼ cup ground cinnamon
2 tablespoons whole cardamom seeds
2 tablespoons whole cloves
1 tablespoon whole cumin seeds
1 tablespoon ground mace
⅛ teaspoon ground nutmeg

Place all ingredients in a small skillet and roast lightly over medium-high heat until the spices darken in color and smell fragrant—about 2 minutes. Grind together in a clean coffee grinder. Store in an airtight bottle away from heat and strong light.

Yield: about 10 tablespoons.

Recipe adapted from *Totally Hot* (Doubleday, 1986), by Michael Goodwin, Charles Perry, and Naomi Wise.

The following preparations for tofu are used in recipes in this book. Nutritional information is given in those recipes.

DEEP-FRIED TOFU

1 package (10½ ounces) firm tofu
3 cups vegetable oil

Cut tofu into 2-inch cubes, or into triangles of about 3 inches per side. Place on several layers of paper towels and let stand several minutes to drain; gently dry with fresh paper towels. Heat oil in large skillet or wok to 375° F. Slide several tofu pieces into oil; do not crowd pan. If they stick together, gently separate them with long chopsticks or two long spoons. Fry until firm and golden all over, turning frequently. Remove with chopsticks or a slotted spoon; drain on a double thickness of paper towels. Repeat with remaining tofu.

Note: For later use, place fried tofu in plastic bag or a covered container and refrigerate for up to 5 days.

GRILLED OR BROILED TOFU CUTLET

1 package (10½ ounces) firm tofu, cut into slices 1 inch thick
1 tablespoon light soy sauce
1 teaspoon dark (Asian) sesame oil

Dry tofu on several layers of paper towels, patting gently. With a pastry brush, brush tofu with combined soy sauce and sesame oil. Cook immediately, or let marinate, refrigerated, several hours.

Grill tofu over medium-hot coals until well-browned, about 5 minutes. Turn; brush with soy mixture, and continue cooking until browned and slightly crisp at the edges.

Tofu can also be broiled, 5 inches from heat source, until browned, about 5 minutes on each side.

If not using immediately, place in a covered container, and refrigerate up to 5 days.

Note: Grilled tofu has a firm, chewy texture and a meaty flavor. Its flavor can be varied by marinating it in other mixtures, such as teriyaki sauce, hoisin sauce, bottled Indian or Southeast Asian curry paste, or barbecue sauce (Western or Chinese).

PLAIN BAKED TOFU CUTLET

1 package (10½ ounces) firm tofu, cut into slices 1 inch thick

Dry tofu on several layers of paper towels, patting gently. Place tofu in ungreased baking pan and bake at 375° F for 20–30 minutes, until firm and dry. Pour off liquid from pan. If not using immediately, store in a covered container, refrigerated, for up to 5 days.

Note: Baked tofu is firm and chewy.

Appetizers, Snacks, & Pick–Me–Ups

★

CHICKPEA DIP (HUMMUS)

PER SERVING: 80 CALORIES, 3.2 G PROTEIN, 7.9 G CARBOHYDRATE, 4.5 G FAT (0.6 G SATURATED),
294.9 MG SODIUM, 2.0 G FIBER, **PE CONTENT 0–5 MG PER CUP**

1 cup cooked chickpeas (garbanzo beans, see page 86)
2–3 cloves garlic
¼ cup tahini (see Glossary of Ingredients, page 82)
¼ cup water
1 teaspoon salt
¼ teaspoon pepper
2–3 tablespoons lemon juice

Process all ingredients in blender or food processor until smooth.

Serve as a dip with raw vegetables, pita bread, and savory crackers, or as a topping for baked potatoes.

Serves 8 (about 3 tablespoons each).

Note: Reduce the amount of garlic in this recipe if garlic on your breath worries you.

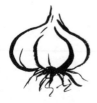

Chickpeas are quite sweet by themselves and have a very nice flavor. Most people can eat them unflavored. Roasted chickpeas are commonly eaten as a savory snack by young and old in Southeast Asian countries.

SOYBEAN DIP

★
★
★

PER SERVING: 50 CALORIES, 3.8 G PROTEIN, 2.6 G CARBOHYDRATE, 3.1 G FAT (0.5 G SATURATED), 292.9 MG SODIUM, 1.4 G FIBER, **PE CONTENT 10–15 MG**

2 teaspoons finely chopped red onion
½ tablespoon olive or soybean oil
1 teaspoon curry powder
2 tablespoons water, divided
¾ cup cooked soybeans (see page 87)
¾ teaspoon salt
1 tablespoon plain, low-fat yogurt

Sauté onion in oil in small skillet 2 minutes on low to medium heat. Stir in curry powder and 1 tablespoon water and sauté 2–3 minutes, until fragrant but not dry.

Process onion mixture and remaining ingredients in food processor or blender until smooth.

Serve as a dip with raw vegetables or crackers. This dip can also be spread on bread and lightly toasted under the broiler.

Serves 6 (about 2 tablespoons each).

If you are using frozen cooked soybeans, rinse them in hot water before using in this recipe.

Although some dips are higher in fat content than other dishes, it is to be noted that these sorts of foods should be eaten in moderation. Low-fat crackers, toasted bread, and vegetables, used as accompaniments, will reduce the overall percentage of fat in relation to the total energy intake.

★

SPICY LENTIL DIP

PER SERVING: 127.0 CALORIES, 8.0 G PROTEIN, 17.3 G CARBOHYDRATE, 3.4 G FAT (0.8 G SATURATED), 139.0 MG SODIUM, 6.6 G FIBER, **PE CONTENT 0–5 MG PER CUP**

½ small onion, finely chopped
1 tablespoon plus 1 teaspoon olive or soybean oil
1 red chili, seeded, finely chopped
1 teaspoon finely chopped gingerroot
1 cup dry lentils, rinsed, sorted
½ teaspoon ground cumin
¼ teaspoon ground turmeric
1½ cups Asian-Style Chicken Stock (see page 88)
or canned reduced-sodium chicken broth
½ teaspoon garam masala (see page 89)
½ teaspoon salt
2 tablespoons finely shredded unsweetened coconut

Sauté onion in oil in medium saucepan until lightly browned, about 4 minutes. Add chili and gingerroot; sauté 2 minutes longer. Add lentils, cumin, and turmeric; cook 2–3 minutes. Stir in stock; heat to boiling. Reduce heat and simmer, covered, 20 minutes. Stir in remaining ingredients; simmer, covered, until lentils are tender, about 15 minutes. Cool. Process in food processor until smooth.

Serve cold with raw vegetables or savory crackers.

Serves 8 (about 3 tablespoons each).

Notes: If you do not wish to make your own, prepared garam masala is available at East Indian groceries and by mail order.

The lentils can also be served hot; do not puree. Spoon over steamed rice.

Lentils are rich in fiber, proteins, iron, and potassium. This legume also contains phytoestrogens.

SPRING ROLLS ★

PER SERVING: 275 CALORIES, 11.2 G PROTEIN, 43.4 G CARBOHYDRATE, 6.1 G FAT (1.8 G SATURATED), 768.5 MG SODIUM, 3.0 G FIBER, **PE CONTENT 0–5 MG PER RECIPE**

7 ounces ground pork (see Glossary of Ingredients, page 81,
and note, page 98)
1 tablespoon plus 1 teaspoon light soy sauce
1 tablespoon plus 1 teaspoon oyster sauce
2 teaspoons vegetable oil
1 clove garlic, minced
5¾ cups shredded cabbage
¾ cup bamboo shoots, cut into strips
1¼ cups diced carrots
1 can (5 ounces) bean sprouts, rinsed, drained
10 stalks garlic chives, or chives, cut into 2-inch lengths
1 teaspoon salt
Pinch pepper
1 tablespoon plus 1 teaspoon cornstarch
⅓ cup water
20 frozen spring-roll wrappers (8 x 8–inch sheets)
1 egg white, lightly beaten

Combine pork, soy sauce, and oyster sauce in small bowl.

Heat 2 teaspoons oil in wok or large skillet over medium heat until hot. Stir-fry garlic in oil until fragrant, about 1 minute; add pork mixture and stir-fry until lightly browned, about 3 minutes. Increase heat to high; add cabbage, bamboo shoots, and carrots. Stir-fry until cabbage is wilted, about 2 minutes; add bean sprouts, chives, salt, and pepper. Stir-fry 1 minute; drain in metal colander and cool.

Mix cornstarch and water in small microwave-safe bowl; microwave on high until thickened, about 30 seconds.

Defrost spring-roll wrappers following package directions. Divide filling into 20 portions and wrap in spring-roll wrappers, tucking in ends of wrapper as you roll. Seal edges with cornstarch paste.

Brush wrappers with lightly beaten egg whites. Bake on lightly greased cookie sheet at 325° F for 30 minutes, or until browned.

Serve hot with Chinese mustard, ketchup, plum sauce, or sweet and sour sauce.

Makes 10 servings of 2 rolls each.

Note: Those who do not wish to use pork can substitute ground chicken breast in this recipe, and this change will reduce the overall fat content. Homemade spring rolls are special treats and are suitable for special occasions. Vegetarians can use deep-fried tofu (tofu buk); shred it into strips with a sharp knife before adding it to the recipe. Adding tofu will boost the PE content of this dish.

GRILLED SOY CHEESE SANDWICHES

★
★
★
★

PER SERVING: 240 CALORIES, 13.7 G PROTEIN, 25.6 G CARBOHYDRATE, 10.5 G FAT (3.3 G SATURATED), 476.0 MG SODIUM, 2.5 G FIBER, **PE CONTENT 10–15 MG**

2 slices Crusty Soy Bread (see page 200), or whole-grain bread
1 teaspoon butter or margarine
⅓ cup alfalfa sprouts, divided
1 tablespoon plus 1 teaspoon shredded carrot
¼ cup (1 ounce) grated soy cheese
Salt and pepper, to taste
Cherry tomatoes, as garnish

Spread top of bread thinly with butter or margarine. Place 1 slice of bread, buttered side down, in small skillet. Top with ¼ cup alfalfa sprouts, carrot, and soy cheese. Sprinkle lightly with salt and pepper. Cover with second slice of bread, buttered side up. Cook over low heat until brown on 1 side; turn and cook on second side until golden brown.

Slice the sandwich in half; garnish with remaining alfalfa sprouts and cherry tomatoes.

Serves 1.

Note: Sandwich can also be cooked in a sandwich grill or waffle iron, following manufacturer's instructions.

Alfalfa sprouts are a rich source of lignans, coumestans (chemicals that have an estrogenic effect), and vitamin C. As fresh sprouts are very lightweight, a package will last for a few meals. A few people dislike sprouts' green, beany taste, but this almost disappears when they're cooked inside a sandwich.

★
★
★
★
★
+

Soy-Banana Breakfast Drink

PER DRINK: 270 CALORIES, 5.4 G PROTEIN, 45.7 G CARBOHYDRATE, 8.9 G FAT (2.1 G SATURATED), 192.2 MG SODIUM, 1.8 G FIBER, **PE CONTENT 15–20 MG PER CUP**

1 cup soy milk, chilled
1 ripe banana, sliced
1–2 teaspoons sugar
¼ teaspoon vanilla extract (optional)

Process all ingredients in blender or food processor until smooth. Serves 1 (about 1½ cups).

Commercially prepared soy milk is readily available. The UHT (ultra heat treated) or long-life soy milk tastes different from homemade soy milk. Some preparations are fat-reduced, and these are particularly good for people on a weight-reduction diet. Some brands are calcium-enriched and therefore good for those who need more dietary calcium. Some brands of soy milk are already flavored and come in 8-fluid-ounce UHT packages, making them convenient for lunch or picnic packs. Soy milk made from whole beans also tastes different from those reconstituted with soy protein and other additives.

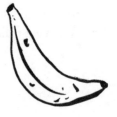

Avoid bananas if you suffer from reflux problems or joint pains, as they may aggravate the condition. Cantaloupe, mangoes, peaches, and strawberries are good alternatives to bananas.

CANTALOUPE-SOY MILK SHAKE

★
★
★
★
★
+

PER SERVING: 176 CALORIES, 8.0 G PROTEIN, 30.9 G CARBOHYDRATE, 3.2 G FAT (0.1 G SATURATED), 48.5 MG SODIUM, 1.8 G FIBER, **PE CONTENT OVER 25 MG**

2 cups diced cantaloupe
1 tablespoon plus 1 teaspoon honey
½ cup low-fat soy milk, chilled
7 ounces silken tofu, chilled

Process all the ingredients in blender or food processor until smooth. Chill before serving.

Serves 2 (about 1½ cups each).

Cantaloupes are rich in beta-carotene, a compound linked to lower lung cancer rates. The melons also have blood-thinning properties, as they inhibit platelet aggregation and thus reduce the risk of blood clots forming within blood vessels.

★
★
★
★
★
+

STRAWBERRY SOY DRINK

PER SERVING: 153 CALORIES, 4.7 G PROTEIN, 30.6 G CARBOHYDRATE, 2.4 G FAT (0.0 G SATURATED),
91.2 MG SODIUM, 4.5 G FIBER, **PE CONTENT 20–25 MG PER CUP**

1 cup low-fat soy milk, chilled
2–3 teaspoons sugar
¾ cup sliced strawberries

Process all ingredients in blender or food processor until smooth.
Chill before serving.

Serves 1 (about 1¾ cups).

TROPICAL FRUIT SMOOTHIE

★
★
★
★
★
+

PER SERVING: 222 CALORIES, 5.0 G PROTEIN, 33.2 G CARBOHYDRATE, 8.8 G FAT (2.0 G SATURATED),
192.1 MG SODIUM, 1.4 G FIBER, **PE CONTENT 15–20 MG PER CUP**

½ cup fresh pineapple chunks
1 ripe banana
¼ teaspoon coconut extract
2 cups vanilla-flavored soy milk
4–6 ice cubes
Pineapple wedge and toasted coconut, as garnish

Blend all ingredients, except pineapple wedge and coconut, in
blender or food processor until smooth. Pour into glasses; garnish with
pineapple wedge and coconut.

Serves 2 (about 1½ cups each).

Recipe from *Healthy and Delicious Recipes, Vol. 1.* By permission of VitaSoy.

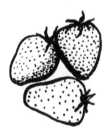

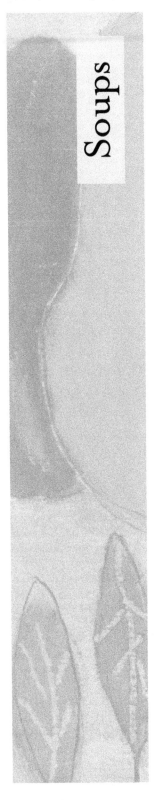

Soups

★
★
★
★
★
+

MISO SOUP

PER SERVING: 167 CALORIES, 14.4 G PROTEIN, 11.7 G CARBOHYDRATE, 8.1 G FAT (1.3 G SATURATED),
997.1 MG SODIUM, 3.8 G FIBER **PE CONTENT OVER 25 MG**

1 cup plus 2 tablespoons water, divided
Dashi stock paste
(or concentrate, if using plain miso paste; see Glossary of Ingredients, page 80)
1 green onion, green parts only, cut into ¾-inch lengths
3½ ounces firm tofu, cut into ½-inch cubes
1 level tablespoon plus 1 level teaspoon miso paste
(see Glossary of Ingredients, page 81)

Heat 1 cup water and dashi stock to boiling in small saucepan;
reduce heat and simmer, uncovered, 3 minutes. Add green onion and
tofu. Dissolve miso paste in remaining 2 tablespoons water in small
bowl; stir into soup. Stir over medium heat until hot.

Serves 1.

Note: Firm tofu is normally used in this recipe, but many people
prefer the soup with smooth, tender silken tofu instead.

Miso soup is a popular Japanese breakfast dish.
Dashi paste is available from Asian food stores and
the Asian food sections of large supermarkets.

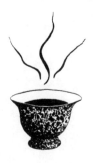

CREAMY CORN SOUP ★ ★

PER SERVING: 135 CALORIES, 10.8 G PROTEIN, 17.6 G CARBOHYDRATE, 2.8 G FAT (0.3 G SATURATED), 506.0 MG SODIUM, 0.9 G FIBER, **PE CONTENT 5–10 MG**

2 tablespoons plus 2 teaspoons cornstarch, divided
1 tablespoon plus 1 teaspoon light soy sauce
2 ounces skinless, boneless chicken breast, cut into thin strips
4 cups Asian-Style Chicken Stock (see page 88),
or canned reduced-sodium chicken broth
1 can (15½ ounces) cream-style corn
5 ounces silken tofu
¼ cup water
1 egg
Salt, to taste

Combine 2 teaspoons cornstarch and soy sauce in small bowl. Add the chicken strips and toss to coat; marinate at least 10 minutes.

Heat stock to boiling in large saucepan. Stir in chicken mixture; reduce heat and simmer 5 minutes. Stir in corn.

Process tofu, water, and egg in blender or food processor until smooth; stir into soup. Heat over medium heat until hot and slightly thickened. If you prefer a thicker, glossier soup, mix remaining 2 tablespoons cornstarch with small amount of cold water, and use to thicken soup. Season to taste with salt.

Serves 6.

This is a very creamy and tasty recipe. Omit the tofu if you do not enjoy a creamy taste. A very tasty variation of this soup substitutes crabmeat for chicken. (Add the crabmeat just a minute before adding the tofu.) In West Africa, a spicy version is popular: substitute chopped raw shrimp or prawns for the chicken, and stir in cayenne or hot sauce until the soup is quite spicy. The African version can be made with water instead of stock for pisco-vegetarians. Both the corn and tofu in this recipe contain phytoestrogens. Omit the egg if you are on a low-cholesterol diet.

★
★

TOMATO CORN CHOWDER

PER SERVING: 134 CALORIES, 4.9 G PROTEIN, 21.5 G CARBOHYDRATE, 4.2 G FAT (0.5 G SATURATED),
378.5 MG SODIUM, 4.1 G FIBER, **PE CONTENT 5–10 MG**

1 onion, chopped
1 tablespoon vegetable oil
2 carrots, cut in half lengthwise and sliced
2 ribs celery, thinly sliced
1–2 cloves garlic, mashed
2 cups water, or canned vegetable broth
2 medium potatoes, peeled, diced
¾ to 1 cup fresh or thawed, frozen whole kernel corn
2 tablespoons soy sauce
1 teaspoon dried, or 1 tablespoon chopped fresh basil
1 bay leaf
2 roma tomatoes, peeled, seeded, diced
2 cups soy milk
Salt and black pepper, to taste
Cayenne pepper, to taste
Grated Parmesan cheese, as garnish

Sauté onion in oil in large saucepan until tender, about 3 minutes; stir in carrots, celery, and garlic and sauté 2–3 minutes.

Add water, potatoes, corn, soy sauce, and herbs. Heat to boiling; reduce heat and simmer until potatoes are soft, about 15 minutes.

Add tomatoes and soy milk; heat to simmering. Season to taste with salt, black pepper, and cayenne pepper. Serve with a sprinkle of cheese on top.

Serves 6.

Recipe from *Healthy and Delicious Recipes, Vol. 1.* By permission of VitaSoy.

CREAMY TOMATO SOUP

★
★
★
★
★
+

PER SERVING: 117 CALORIES, 8.4 G PROTEIN, 11.6 G CARBOHYDRATE, 4.7 G FAT (0.6 G SATURATED), 505.6 MG SODIUM, 1.9 G FIBER, **PE CONTENT OVER 25 MG**

1 medium onion, diced
2 teaspoons vegetable oil
1 large tomato, diced
½ teaspoon chopped garlic
1 cup low-fat soy milk
1 teaspoon chopped fresh basil
½ teaspoon salt
½ teaspoon white pepper
1 package (10½ ounces) low-fat, firm silken tofu

Sauté onion in oil in medium saucepan until tender, about 3 minutes. Add tomato and garlic and sauté 2–3 minutes. Add soy milk, basil, salt, and pepper. Cook over medium-high heat, stirring constantly, for 1 minute. Remove from heat and cool briefly.

Process soup and tofu in blender or food processor until smooth. Serve hot or chilled.

Serves 3.

Recipe courtesy of the Indiana Soybean Board.

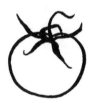

★
★

CREAMY PUMPKIN SOUP

PER SERVING: 94 CALORIES, 5.2 G PROTEIN, 15.8 G CARBOHYDRATE, 1.9 G FAT (0.2 G SATURATED), 79.6 MG SODIUM, 2.6 G FIBER, **PE CONTENT 5–10 MG**

1 pound pumpkin, peeled, seeded, diced
1 medium apple, peeled, diced
1 medium potato, peeled, diced
1 medium onion, peeled, diced
1⅔ cups Asian-Style Chicken Stock (see page 88),
or canned reduced-sodium chicken or vegetable broth
1⅔ cups soy milk
1 tablespoon plus 1 teaspoon cornstarch (optional)
Salt and pepper, to taste
Parsley sprigs, as garnish

Combine pumpkin, apple, potato, onion, and stock in large saucepan. Heat to boiling; reduce heat and simmer, covered, until tender, about 20 minutes.

Process soup in blender or food processor until smooth; return soup to pan. Add soy milk and heat to boiling.

If you prefer a thicker, glossier soup, mix cornstarch with 2 teaspoons water and add to soup, stirring until slightly thickened. Season to taste with salt and pepper. Garnish with parsley.

Serves 6.

The pumpkin, apple, and potato in this recipe all contain phytoestrogens. If a creamier soup is desired, replace the soy milk with 5 ounces silken tofu blended into a smooth purée with 1⅔ cups water or broth.

Lentil-Vegetable Soup ★

PER SERVING: 207 CALORIES, 16.3 G PROTEIN, 30.2 G CARBOHYDRATE, 2.5 G FAT (0.1 G SATURATED), 347.1 MG SODIUM, 8.3 G FIBER, **PE CONTENT 0–5 MG**

½ cup red lentils
¼ cup pearl barley
8 cups Asian-Style Chicken Stock (see page 88),
or canned reduced-sodium chicken or vegetable broth
2 large potatoes, diced
1 carrot, diced
3 tomatoes, diced
1 onion, diced
Salt and pepper, to taste
Chopped parsley, as garnish

Combine lentils, barley, and stock in large saucepan; heat to boiling. Reduce heat and simmer, covered, ½ hour. Add the potatoes, carrot, tomatoes, and onion. Heat to boiling; reduce heat and simmer, covered, until barley and vegetables are tender, about 40 minutes. Season to taste with salt and pepper. Garnish with parsley.

Serves 6.

Celery can substitute for onions and tomatoes. Packaged soup mixes containing pearl barley, split peas, lentils, etc., can be used instead of lentils and pearl barley. The red lentils, pearl barley, carrots, and potatoes in this recipe all contain phytoestrogens.

★
★

CREAMY POTATO SOUP

PER SERVING: 292 CALORIES, 7.3 G PROTEIN, 46.8 G CARBOHYDRATE, 9.2 G FAT (1.1 G SATURATED), 350.5 MG SODIUM, 5.7 G FIBER, **PE CONTENT 5–10 MG**

1 onion, diced
2–3 carrots, diced
2 medium potatoes, peeled, diced
3 tablespoons vegetable oil
1 tablespoon dried dill weed
2 teaspoons minced garlic
4 cups canned reduced-sodium vegetable broth
2¼ cups soy milk
1 cup instant mashed potatoes
Salt and white pepper, to taste
Grated Parmesan, Swiss, or Cheddar cheese (optional)

Sauté onion, carrots, and potatoes in oil in large saucepan until onion is translucent, about 5 minutes. Add dill and garlic, and sauté 2–3 minutes. Add broth; heat to boiling. Reduce heat and simmer, covered, until potatoes are tender, about 15 minutes. Add soy milk and instant potatoes, stirring thoroughly to blend; stir over medium heat until hot. Season to taste with salt and white pepper. Sprinkle with cheese if desired.

Serves 6.

Recipe from *Healthy and Delicious Recipes, Vol. 1*. By permission of VitaSoy.

CURRIED CARROT SOUP ★

PER SERVING: 85 CALORIES, 3.4 G PROTEIN, 15.2 G CARBOHYDRATE, 1.7 G FAT (0.4 G SATURATED),
453.8 MG SODIUM, 3.9 G FIBER, **PE CONTENT 0–5 MG**

6 medium carrots, sliced
2 cups canned reduced-sodium vegetable broth
1 small onion, chopped
2 teaspoons curry powder
½ cup soy milk

Combine all ingredients, except soy milk, in large saucepan. Heat
to boiling; reduce heat and simmer, covered, until carrots are tender,
about 20 minutes. Process in blender or food processor until smooth;
return to saucepan. Stir in soy milk. Cook over low heat until hot.
Serves 4.

Recipe courtesy of the Indiana Soybean Board.

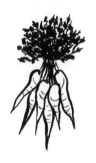

★
★
★
★
★

TOFU AND WATERCRESS SOUP

PER SERVING: 71 CALORIES, 8.7 G PROTEIN, 2.6 G CARBOHYDRATE, 2.4 G FAT (0.0 G SATURATED),
596.1 MG SODIUM, 0.3 G FIBER, **PE CONTENT 20–25 MG**

1 large bunch (½ pound) watercress
2 cups boiling water
2 cups canned reduced-sodium chicken or vegetable broth
2 teaspoons chicken or vegetable bouillon crystals
10 ounces silken tofu, drained, cut into ½-inch cubes
Salt and pepper, to taste

Wash watercress and remove any yellow leaves. Separate tough stems from tender leaves and stems. Cut tender leaves and stems into ½-inch pieces.

Add tough watercress stems to boiling water in medium saucepan. Reduce heat and simmer, covered, 20 minutes; remove stems and discard. Heat to boiling. Stir in cut watercress, broth, and bouillon. Simmer until watercress is tender, about 3 minutes. Add tofu, and stir just until soup is warm. Season to taste with salt and pepper.

Serves 4.

Note: Watercress may taste bitter if added before the water has boiled.

HEALTHY POTATO LEEK SOUP

★
★

PER SERVING: 131 CALORIES, 3.7 G PROTEIN, 22.0 G CARBOHYDRATE, 3.3 G FAT (0.2 G SATURATED), 321.0 MG SODIUM, 2.2 G FIBER, **PE CONTENT 5–10 MG**

10 ounces leeks, white parts only, sliced
1 tablespoon vegetable oil (canola, peanut, or soy)
12 ounces peeled, cubed potatoes
4 cups Asian-Style Chicken Stock (see page 88), or canned vegetable broth
5 ounces silken tofu, cubed
Salt and pepper, to taste

Sauté leeks in oil in medium saucepan until soft and fragrant, about 4 minutes. Stir in potatoes and stock. Heat to boiling; reduce heat and simmer, covered, until potatoes are tender, about 20 minutes. Stir in tofu. Process in blender or food processor until smooth. Season to taste with salt and pepper. Heat to simmering; do not boil.

Serves 6.

★
★
★
★
★

SEAFOOD TOFU SOUP

PER SERVING: 194 CALORIES, 19.9 G PROTEIN, 16.5 G CARBOHYDRATE, 5.3 G FAT (0.8 G SATURATED),
609.8 MG SODIUM, 2.2 G FIBER, **PE CONTENT 20–25 MG**

1 ounce dried shiitake (Chinese black) mushrooms
Hot water, for soaking mushrooms
6 ounces shrimp, lean white fish fillets, or other seafood, cut into ¾-inch cubes
1 tablespoon light soy sauce
1 tablespoon cornstarch
Dash pepper
4 ounces thinly sliced leeks, white parts only
1 teaspoon vegetable oil
4 thin slices gingerroot
4 ounces sliced carrot
4 cups fish stock, clam juice, or vegetable broth
10 ounces silken tofu, cut into ½-inch cubes
Lime slices, as garnish

In a small bowl, soak dried mushrooms in hot water to cover until softened, about 10 minutes. Remove tough stems and discard; slice tops thinly.

Combine seafood, soy sauce, cornstarch, and pepper in small bowl.

Sauté leeks in oil in medium saucepan until tender, about 3 minutes. Add ginger, carrot, and mushrooms. Sauté 3 minutes, or until lightly browned. Add stock and heat to boiling; reduce heat and simmer until vegetables are tender, about 10 minutes. Add seafood and simmer 4–5 minutes, until seafood is cooked through. Stir in tofu; heat to boiling and remove from heat.

Ladle soup into bowls; garnish with lime slices.

Serves 4.

Split Pea and Carrot Soup ★

PER SERVING: 316 CALORIES, 21.7 G PROTEIN, 49.8 G CARBOHYDRATE, 4.0 G FAT (0.4 G SATURATED), 603.5 MG SODIUM, 20.0 G FIBER, **PE CONTENT 0–5 MG**

1 ½ cups dried yellow split peas
3 cups hot water, for soaking
Pinch baking soda
½ cup chopped onion
1–2 teaspoons chopped gingerroot
2 teaspoons vegetable oil
6 ounces chopped carrots
2 ounces chopped celery
3 cups boiling water
2 cups canned reduced-sodium chicken or vegetable broth
2 teaspoons chicken or vegetable bouillon crystals
1 ounce diced low-fat ham (optional)
Salt and pepper, to taste
Parsley, as garnish

Combine split peas, hot water, and baking soda in medium bowl; let soak several hours or overnight. Drain and rinse before using.

Sauté onion and gingerroot in oil in large saucepan until soft, about 3 minutes. Add carrots, celery, drained split peas, and boiling water. Heat to boiling; reduce heat and simmer 30 minutes. Add broth, bouillon, and ham, if using. Simmer, covered, until split peas are tender, about 10 minutes.

Process in food processor or blender until smooth. Return soup to saucepan and heat to boiling; season to taste with salt and pepper. Sprinkle with parsley.

Serves 4.

Salads, Dressings, & Side Dishes

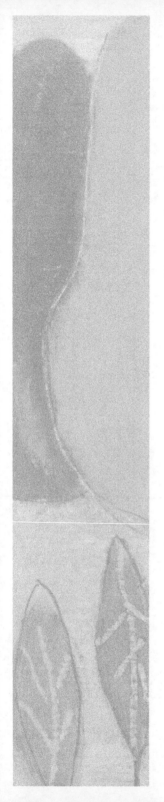

CHICKPEA SALAD ★

PER SERVING: 109 CALORIES, 4.4 G PROTEIN, 14.6 G CARBOHYDRATE, 4.2 G FAT (0.5 G SATURATED), 319.8 MG SODIUM, 3.7 G FIBER, **PE CONTENT 0–5 MG**

1½ cups cooked or canned chickpeas (garbanzo beans),
rinsed, drained (see page 86)
1 large, or 2 medium tomatoes, diced
½ cup diced celery
6 stalks chives, finely chopped
2 fresh basil leaves, finely chopped
Garlic Dressing (recipe follows)
Salt and pepper, to taste

Combine all ingredients, except salt and pepper, in large bowl. Toss well; season to taste with salt and pepper.

Serve with roasted chicken or barbecue, or as part of a vegetarian salad assortment.

Serves 6.

GARLIC DRESSING

(makes about ¼ cup)

2 cloves garlic, sliced
1 tablespoon plus 1 teaspoon olive or canola oil
¼ teaspoon pepper
¼ teaspoon ground cinnamon
½ teaspoon salt
1 teaspoon sugar
1 tablespoon plus 1 teaspoon lemon juice
1 tablespoon plus 1 teaspoon light soy sauce

Sauté garlic in oil in small skillet until golden brown. Discard garlic; set oil aside until cool.

Shake garlic oil and remaining ingredients in glass jar with lid.

★
★
★
★

BEAN SALAD

PER SERVING: 124 CALORIES, 6.8 G PROTEIN, 17.1 G CARBOHYDRATE, 3.8 G FAT (0.6 G SATURATED), 462.9 MG SODIUM, 4.7 G FIBER, **PE CONTENT 15–20 MG**

1 can or jar (14 ounces) three-bean salad
1 cup cooked soybeans (see page 87)
1 cup cut green beans, cooked crisp-tender, cooled
2 teaspoons finely chopped red bell pepper
2 teaspoons finely chopped onion
½ tablespoon olive oil
1 tablespoon wine vinegar
2 teaspoons sugar
½ teaspoon salt
¼ teaspoon ground cinnamon
¼ teaspoon ground nutmeg
¼ teaspoon pepper

Drain the three-bean salad and rinse with cool water. Place in large bowl with soybeans and green beans. Whisk remaining ingredients in small bowl; pour over bean mixture and toss well. Refrigerate, covered, until serving time; toss well before serving.

Serve cold at picnics, barbecues, or with vegetarian dinner platters. Serves 6.

THAI SALAD

PER SERVING: 159 CALORIES, 11.6 G PROTEIN, 16.3 G CARBOHYDRATE, 6.2 G FAT (0.3 G SATURATED), 1,200.6 MG SODIUM, 3.7 G FIBER, **PE CONTENT 10–15 MG**

5 ounces leaf or romaine lettuce, torn
½ cup chopped cucumber
⅓ cup chopped red bell pepper
1 cup fresh bean sprouts
6 cherry tomatoes, halved
3½ ounces low-fat, hard tofu, cut into small cubes and grilled until light brown
Thai Dressing (recipe follows)
2 tablespoons chopped peanuts, as garnish
Fresh cilantro leaves, as garnish

Arrange lettuce on platter; top with vegetables and grilled tofu. Pour Thai Dressing over salad; garnish with peanuts and cilantro. Serves 4.

THAI DRESSING

(makes about ⅔ cup)

¼ cup nam pla (Thai fish sauce; see note below)
2 tablespoons plus 2 teaspoons boiling water
2 tablespoons plus 2 teaspoons lime juice
1 tablespoon plus 1 teaspoon rice wine vinegar or apple cider vinegar
2 teaspoons olive, peanut, or canola oil
1 tablespoon plus 1 teaspoon chopped fresh cilantro
1 clove garlic, finely chopped
1 small fresh hot red chili, diced
1 tablespoon sugar
½ teaspoon salt

Whisk all ingredients in small bowl. Refrigerate until serving time.

Note: Thai fish sauce can be found in the Asian-food section of most grocery stores. This is an important ingredient for the dressing and gives the salad a unique taste.

★

APPLE AND POTATO SALAD

PER SERVING: 96 CALORIES, 1.4 G PROTEIN, 13.9 G CARBOHYDRATE, 4.4 G FAT (0.9 G SATURATED), 391.3 MG SODIUM, 1.6 G FIBER, **PE CONTENT 0–5 MG**

1 pound small red potatoes
1 large green apple
1 tablespoon plus 1 teaspoon lime juice
1 tablespoonful minced lean ham, or any soy-based smoked "meat"
4–5 stalks fresh chives, snipped
½ cup thinly sliced celery
6 tablespoons plus 2 teaspoons light mayonnaise
or Tofu Mayonnaise (see page 131)

1 teaspoon salt
½ teaspoon pepper

Cook potatoes in boiling water in medium saucepan until tender, about 12 minutes. Drain; cool. Cut into ¾-inch cubes.

Cut apple into ¾-inch cubes and toss with lime juice in large bowl. Add potatoes and remaining ingredients and toss well. Refrigerate, covered, until chilled, about 1 hour.

Serves 8.

Note: Diced cooked chicken breast can be used instead of ham in this recipe. Vegetarians may replace the meat with walnuts, pistachios, or sunflower seeds.

Apples contain **estrone**, which is a natural estrogen that circulates in the blood of post-menopausal women. Other foods, including rice, also contain estrone, as well as estradiol. **Estradiol** predominantly circulates in the blood of premenopausal women. Pomegranates contain estrone, too; hence their Chinese nickname, the "fertility fruit."

Soy Macaroni Salad

★
★

PER SERVING: 212 CALORIES, 6.7 G PROTEIN, 29.9 G CARBOHYDRATE, 7.8 G FAT (1.6 G SATURATED), 430.9 MG SODIUM, 2.8 G FIBER, **PE CONTENT 5–10 MG**

7 ounces soy macaroni, cooked, cooled
1 cup frozen green peas, thawed
1 tablespoonful minced lean ham
2 teaspoons finely chopped onion
¼ cup shredded carrot
¼ teaspoon salt
¼ teaspoon sugar
½ cup light mayonnaise or Tofu Mayonnaise (see page 131)
Ground black pepper, to taste
1 tablespoon grated Parmesan cheese (optional)

Combine all ingredients, except pepper and cheese, in medium bowl; season to taste with pepper. Refrigerate at least 1 hour before serving. Sprinkle with cheese.

Serve at picnics or barbecues. A green salad complements this dish very nicely.

Serves 6.

★
★
★
★

GREEK TOFU SALAD

PER SERVING: 105 CALORIES, 7.7 G PROTEIN, 4.5 G CARBOHYDRATE, 6.7 G FAT (1.1 G SATURATED), 305.7 MG SODIUM, 0.9 G FIBER, **PE CONTENT 15–20 MG**

¼ cup sun-dried tomatoes (not oil packed)
Hot water
1½ teaspoons dried oregano leaves
1 teaspoon olive oil
1 tablespoon red wine vinegar
12 pitted kalamata olives, each cut into 3 pieces
1 tablespoon chopped red onion
10 ounces extra-firm tofu, drained, cut into ½-inch cubes
⅔ cup cubed seedless (English) cucumber (½-inch cubes)
1 tablespoon chopped parsley
Salt and pepper, to taste
Boston or Bibb lettuce leaves, as garnish

Barely cover tomatoes with hot water in small bowl; let stand 20 minutes. Drain and reserve soaking water. Chop tomatoes.

Mix 1 tablespoon tomato soaking water, oregano, olive oil, red wine vinegar, sun-dried tomatoes, olives, and onion in serving bowl. Add tofu and gently toss to mix. Refrigerate, covered, 1 to 2 hours for flavors to blend.

Just before serving, add cucumber and parsley; mix well. Season to taste with salt and pepper. Line 4 plates with lettuce leaves. Spoon salad on lettuce.

Serves 4.

Recipe adapted from *Delicious and Easy Recipes for Tofu and Pasta*. By permission of Azumaya.

GREEN SOYBEAN SALAD

★
★
★
★

PER SERVING: 184 CALORIES, 15.4 G PROTEIN, 4.4 G CARBOHYDRATE, 8.9 G FAT (1.3 G SATURATED), 112.0 MG SODIUM, 4.9 G FIBER, **PE CONTENT 10–15 MG**

2 cups fresh green soybeans, boiled in lightly salted water for 4 minutes
½ cup finely chopped celery
¼ cup chopped green bell pepper
1 large tomato, diced
⅓ cup low-fat salad dressing (such as French, Italian, or ranch)
Lettuce

Cool boiled green soybeans before use.

Combine all ingredients, except lettuce, in large bowl. Toss well; serve on a bed of lettuce.

Serves 4.

Recipe courtesy of the Indiana Soybean Board.

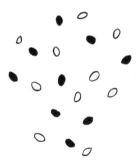

★

SUMMERTIME PICKLED CURRIED VEGETABLES

PER SERVING: 96 CALORIES, 3.1 G PROTEIN, 12.0 G CARBOHYDRATE, 5.0 G FAT (0.7 G SATURATED), 1,183.5 MG SODIUM, 3.5 G FIBER, **PE CONTENT 0–5 MG**

1 medium carrot, cut into 2-inch strips
5 cups sliced cabbage
4 cups cauliflower florets
½ cup cut green beans
3 long red chilies (such as Numex, Italian frying peppers, or Anaheim),
cut into strips
2 cucumbers, cut into 2-inch strips
3 tablespoons curry powder
¼ cup water
1 medium onion, finely chopped
2 tablespoons vegetable oil (soy, peanut, canola)
¾ cup white or apple cider vinegar
2 tablespoons sugar
2 tablespoons salt
8 cloves garlic, quartered
¼ cup finely chopped roasted peanuts
2 tablespoons toasted sesame seeds

Arrange carrot, cabbage, cauliflower, green beans, chilies, and cucumbers in single layer on baking sheets. Place in the sun for at least 4 hours to semi-dry the vegetables. Cover with a food screen or cheesecloth to protect food from pests. The vegetables are ready when they look wrinkled and feel dry to the touch.

Combine curry powder and water in small bowl to make smooth paste.

Cook onion in oil in wok or large skillet over high heat 1 minute; add curry paste and reduce heat to medium. Stir until the mixture is very fragrant, about 1 minute; add vinegar, sugar, and salt.

Increase heat to high, and add carrot, cabbage, and cauliflower. Stir over high heat until cabbage is wilted, about 4 minutes. Add beans and garlic. Heat to boiling; add chilies and cucumber. Heat to boiling, stirring constantly; immediately transfer to shallow dish and cool. Refrigerate, covered, 1–2 days, or up to 1 week.

Before serving, sprinkle with peanuts and sesame seeds.

This spicy relish is good with satay, teriyaki chicken, or any barbecue or picnic food.

Serves 12.

Note: If there is no sun, you can blanch vegetables in boiling water for 30 seconds and then cool them quickly in ice-cold water. Then, place them in cheesecloth so you can hand wring the water out of the vegetables.

The vegetables listed above are those commonly used in this dish. However, if one of the vegetables is out of season, you can simply omit it from the recipe.

This vegetarian dish will delight your taste buds with sweet, sour, savory, hot, and spicy flavors, and it offers a varied texture to accompany your main meal or barbecues.

This dish is prepared a few days ahead of time and stored in the refrigerator until ready to use. The sauce needs a few days to infuse into the vegetables and "pickle" them. This dish is always served cold.

★
★
★

CABBAGE ROLLS

PER ROLL: 179 CALORIES, 9.0 G PROTEIN, 20.8 G CARBOHYDRATE, 6.3 G FAT (1.3 G SATURATED), 699.2 MG SODIUM, 1.9 G FIBER, **PE CONTENT 10–15 MG**

6 large cabbage leaves
1 medium onion, chopped
2 ounces mushrooms, coarsely chopped
½ tablespoon vegetable oil
4 ounces ground meat (chicken, beef, lamb)
2 tablespoons Worcestershire sauce
¼ teaspoon ground black pepper
2 teaspoons beef, chicken, or vegetable bouillon crystals
10 ounces low-fat silken tofu, mashed
½ cup shredded carrots
1½ cups cooked rice
1 can (10¾ ounces) cream of mushroom soup
½ cup water

Preheat oven to 375° F.

Cook cabbage leaves in large pot of boiling water until slightly wilted, about 3 minutes. Drain; remove tough center vein with sharp knife.

Sauté onion and mushrooms in oil until tender, about 5 minutes. Add meat, Worcestershire sauce, pepper, and bouillon; cook until browned, about 5 minutes. Stir in tofu, carrots, and rice.

Wrap meat mixture in cabbage leaves, tucking in sides and securing end with wooden toothpick. Arrange cabbage rolls in lightly greased 9 x 9–inch baking dish. Whisk soup and water together in small bowl until smooth; pour over cabbage rolls. Bake, covered, at 375° F until very tender, about 1 hour.

Serve hot with steamed or roasted vegetables.

Makes 6 rolls.

TOFU MAYONNAISE

★
★
★
★
★
+

PER TABLESPOON: 21 CALORIES, 0.71 G PROTEIN, 0.6 G CARBOHYDRATE, 1.8 G FAT (0.2 G SATURATED), 100.4 MG SODIUM, 0.0 G FIBER, **PE CONTENT OVER 25 MG PER ½ CUP**

5 ounces silken tofu
1 tablespoon plus 1 teaspoon boiling water
2 stalks chives
1 tablespoon white vinegar
1 tablespoon plus 1 teaspoon olive oil
1 teaspoon sugar
½ teaspoon salt
½ teaspoon English or other hot mustard

Process all ingredients in blender or food processor for 30 seconds. Scrape down sides of blender, and blend again until smooth.

Transfer mayonnaise to a clean, airtight container and store in the refrigerator until ready to use.

Makes about 12 tablespoons.

Lemon or lime juice can be used in place of the vinegar in this recipe, but vinegar has some preservative properties. Use mayonnaise made with lemon or lime juice on the same day. However, your mayonnaise will keep up to 3 days if made with vinegar. Silken tofu is best for this recipe, and it must be fresh. Vacuum-sealed packs are more likely to be superior.

★
★

CREAMY POPPY SEED DRESSING

PER TABLESPOON: 80 CALORIES, 1.2 G PROTEIN, 4.4 G CARBOHYDRATE, 6.3 G FAT
(0.1 G SATURATED), 121.7 MG SODIUM, 0.2 G FIBER, **PE CONTENT 5–10 MG PER ½ CUP**

1 cup soybean oil
4 ounces soft silken tofu
½ cup honey
½ cup white vinegar
2 tablespoons poppy seeds
1½ teaspoons dry mustard
1¼ teaspoons salt
1 teaspoon paprika
2 tablespoons minced onion

Process all ingredients, except onion, in food processor or blender until smooth. Stir in onion.

Makes 2½ cups [40 tablespoons].

Recipe from *It's Soy Easy…to Cook with Soy*. By permission of the Ohio Soybean Council.

HEALTHY CAESAR SALAD DRESSING

★
★
★
★

PER TABLESPOON: 93 CALORIES, 3.1 G PROTEIN, 0.4 G CARBOHYDRATE, 8.1 G FAT
(0.0 G SATURATED), 13.7 MG SODIUM, 0.1 G FIBER, **PE CONTENT 15–20 MG PER ½ CUP**

½ cup soybean oil
1 teaspoon minced garlic
4 ounces soft silken tofu
1 tablespoon white wine vinegar
1 tablespoon lemon juice
2 teaspoons Dijon mustard
1 teaspoon lemon pepper
⅛ teaspoon Worchestershire sauce

Process all ingredients in food processor or blender until smooth.
Makes 1 cup.

For Caesar salad, just toss romaine lettuce and croutons with this
healthy dressing.

Recipe from *It's Soy Easy...to Cook with Soy*. By permission of the Ohio Soybean Council.

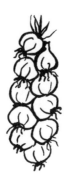

★
★
★

CREAMY BASIL DRESSING

PER TABLESPOON: 37 CALORIES, 0.7 G PROTEIN, 2.1 G CARBOHYDRATE, 2.9 G FAT
(0.5 G SATURATED), 29.9 MG SODIUM, 0.0 G FIBER, **PE CONTENT 10–15 MG PER ½ CUP**

2 cups soy milk
Juice of 1 lemon
1 clove of garlic
6 fresh basil leaves
1 tablespoon olive oil
1 tablespoon vegetable oil
½ teaspoon dried dill weed
¼ teaspoon black pepper
Dash of cayenne pepper
Dash of salt
1 tablespoon grated Parmesan cheese

Process soy milk, lemon juice, garlic, and basil in food processor or blender until smooth; slowly pour in oils while processor is running. Add remaining ingredients, and blend briefly until combined.

Makes about 2 cups.

Recipe from *Healthy and Delicious Recipes, Vol. 1.* By permission of VitaSoy.

CURRIED CHICKPEAS ★

PER SERVING: 167 CALORIES, 5.0 G PROTEIN, 31.4 G CARBOHYDRATE, 3.4 G FAT (0.4 G SATURATED), 607.7 MG SODIUM, 5.2 G FIBER, **PE CONTENT 0–5 MG**

3 ½ ounces dried tamarind or tamarind paste
(or 1 tablespoon bottled tamarind concentrate from India)
½ cup water
1 can (15 ounces) chickpeas, undrained, or 1 ½ cups cooked chickpeas
and ½ cup cooking liquid (see page 86)
1 medium onion, chopped
1 ¾-inch piece gingerroot, finely grated
1 tablespoon vegetable oil
4 green chilies, seeded, chopped
1 teaspoon salt
¼ teaspoon cayenne pepper
1 ½ teaspoons garam masala (see page 89)
Lemon slices, as garnish
½ cup cilantro leaves, chopped, as garnish

Combine dry tamarind or tamarind paste and water in small bowl; soak until softened, about 20 minutes. Remove seeds and pulp; strain and reserve liquid.

Drain chickpeas, reserving liquid.

Sauté onion and ginger in oil in large skillet until lightly browned, about 5 minutes. Add chilies, salt, cayenne, garam masala, and drained chickpeas. Sauté 2–3 minutes, until lightly browned. Stir in reserved tamarind liquid and bean liquid. (If using tamarind concentrate, stir thoroughly to dissolve it with the other ingredients.) Simmer until sauce thickens, about 3 minutes. Spoon into serving dish. Garnish with lemons and sprinkle with cilantro.

Serve hot with steamed rice, pappadams, or chapatis.

Serves 6.

Recipe adapted from an original by Dr. A. Gulati.

Chickpeas contain second-class proteins and phytoestrogens.
Dried tamarind is available in Latin-American and Asian groceries, and tamarind concentrate can be found in East Indian groceries. (Keep the latter refrigerated after opening.) You can substitute 2 tablespoons apple cider vinegar for tamarind in this recipe. Ready-made garam masala is available in East Indian groceries and some regular supermarkets, or from mail-order spice catalogs.

SPICY CHICKPEAS

PER SERVING: 135 CALORIES, 4.6 G PROTEIN, 15.7 G CARBOHYDRATE, 5.8 G FAT (0.8 G SATURATED), 633.4 MG SODIUM, 4.0 G FIBER, **PE CONTENT 5–10 MG**

½ medium onion, diced
1 tablespoon plus 1 teaspoon oil
1 teaspoon garam masala (see page 89)
1 teaspoon cumin seeds
½ teaspoon chili powder
1 tablespoon water
1 can (15 ounces) chickpeas, undrained, or 1½ cups cooked chickpeas
and ½ cup cooking liquid (see page 86)
2 tomatoes, coarsely chopped
2 tablespoons plus 2 teaspoons chopped cilantro
1 teaspoon salt
Cilantro leaves, as garnish

Sauté onion in oil in medium saucepan until translucent, about 3 minutes. Combine garam masala, cumin seeds, chili powder, and water in small bowl to make a paste. Add to onions and sauté until fragrant, about 2 minutes.

Stir in chickpeas and liquid, tomatoes, cilantro, and salt. Heat to boiling; reduce heat and simmer, covered, 10 minutes. Uncover and simmer until thickened, about 5 minutes.

Garnish with cilantro leaves.

Serves 4 to 6.

Recipe adapted from an original by Dr. A. Gulati.

★
★

Soy Samosas

PER SERVING: 175 CALORIES, 6.3 G PROTEIN, 26.5 G CARBOHYDRATE, 4.9 G FAT (0.8 G SATURATED), 272.0 MG SODIUM, 3.3 G FIBER, **PE CONTENT 5–10 MG**

1 ounce chopped onion
1 tablespoon vegetable oil (canola, peanut, soy)
½ teaspoon grated gingerroot
1 teaspoon ground cumin
½ teaspoon ground turmeric
1 cup cooked chickpeas (see page 86) or canned chickpeas
½ cup chickpea cooking liquid or vegetable broth
1 teaspoon vegetable bouillon crystals
4 ounces tofu cutlet or grilled extra-firm tofu (see page 91), finely chopped
1 small potato (about 3 ounces), peeled, cooked, cubed (¼-inch)
½ cup frozen peas, thawed
12 sheets fillo pastry, thawed
Vegetable cooking spray

Sauté onion in oil in small skillet until lightly browned, about 3 minutes. Add gingerroot, cumin, and turmeric, and sauté 1 minute. Mash chickpeas with cooking liquid in medium bowl until coarsely mashed. Stir in onion mixture, bouillon, tofu, potato, and peas. Cool.

Place 1 fillo sheet on counter; spray lightly with cooking spray. Top with 2 more sheets fillo, spraying each with cooking spray. Cut fillo stack into 6 pieces, each about 3 inches wide.

Divide filling into 24 portions, and place one portion at end of fillo strip. Fold fillo over filling, forming a triangle; continue folding back and forth, as if folding a flag. Place on lightly greased baking sheet; repeat with remaining fillo strips and filling. Spray generously with cooking spray.

Bake at 325° F until golden brown, about 20 minutes.

Makes 24 samosas (8 servings of 3 samosas each).

STIR-FRIED GREEN BEANS WITH PINE NUTS

★

PER SERVING: 99 CALORIES, 3.7 G PROTEIN, 10.4 G CARBOHYDRATE, 5.7 G FAT (0.8 G SATURATED), 284.4 MG SODIUM, 4.1 G FIBER, **PE CONTENT 0–5 MG**

1 tablespoon vegetable oil, divided
2 tablespoons pine nuts
1 clove garlic, finely diced
1 pound green beans, cut into 1-inch lengths
1 tablespoon plus 1 teaspoon light soy sauce
1 tablespoon oyster sauce
½ teaspoon cornstarch
¼ cup water
Ground black pepper, to taste

Add 2 drops oil to wok; heat over medium heat until hot. Stir-fry pine nuts until browned, about 3 minutes. Remove pine nuts from wok and drain on paper toweling.

Heat remaining oil in wok over high heat. Stir-fry garlic until lightly browned, about 1 minute; add beans and stir-fry 2–3 minutes. Add soy sauce and oyster sauce. Cook, covered, 1 minute. Stir in combined cornstarch and water; cook until beans are crisp-tender and sauce is thickened, about 3 minutes. Stir in pine nuts; season to taste with pepper.

Serve with steamed rice, pasta, noodles, or meat.

Serves 4.

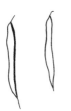

Fresh beans contain coumestrol and lignans. The concentration of coumestrol in fresh green beans is about the same as that in a similar weight of dried soybeans. However, it is 60 to 70 times less than that present in soybean sprouts. The seedling of the green bean is reported to contain estradiol, a natural estrogen found in women's blood.

★
★
★

ASIAN TOFU SALAD

PER SERVING: 215 CALORIES, 12.1 G PROTEIN, 30.0 G CARBOHYDRATE, 7.3 G FAT (0.9 G SATURATED), 803.1 MG SODIUM, 5.9 G FIBER, **PE CONTENT 10–15 MG**

3 cups (6 ounces) mung bean sprouts, stringy ends trimmed
10 ounces firm cooked tofu, cut into ½-inch cubes
1½ cups diagonally cut green beans, cooked crisp-tender, cooled
1 cup julienne carrots
1 medium onion, sliced into thin rings
Thai Lemon Dressing (recipe follows)
2 tablespoons finely chopped roasted peanuts
1 tablespoon lightly toasted sesame seeds

Blanch bean sprouts in boiling water to cover for 20 seconds; drain. Rinse with cold water; drain and pat dry with paper towels. Combine bean sprouts, tofu, beans, carrots, and onion in salad bowl. Add Thai Lemon Dressing and toss. Sprinkle with peanuts and sesame seeds.

Serves 4.

THAI LEMON DRESSING

(makes about ½ cup)

2 tablespoons Thai sweet chili sauce
¼ cup lemon juice
1 tablespoon packed dark brown sugar
1 teaspoon finely chopped lemon grass
½ teaspoon salt
2 tablespoons hot water

Whisk all ingredients in a small bowl.
Serves 4.

Adapted from a recipe provided by Annie Chan.

FIVE SPICED TOFU

★
★
★
★

PER SERVING: 79 CALORIES, 6.3 G PROTEIN, 2.0 G CARBOHYDRATE, 5.2 G FAT (0.6 G SATURATED), 290.7 MG SODIUM, 0.2 G FIBER, **PE CONTENT 15–20 MG**

1 teaspoon Chinese five spice
1 teaspoon white pepper
½ teaspoon salt
½ tablespoon vegetable oil
10 ounces firm tofu

Mix five spice, pepper, and salt and rub evenly over all surfaces of tofu; cut into 2 x 2 x ½–inch pieces.

Heat oil in large nonstick skillet over medium heat until hot. Gently fry tofu until light brown on both sides. Drain on paper towels. Serve as hamburger fillings or on rice with steamed vegetables.

Serves 4.

Adapted from a recipe provided by Annie Chan.

★

BEAN SPROUTS IN FISH SAUCE

PER SERVING: 53 CALORIES, 2.9 G PROTEIN, 6.6 G CARBOHYDRATE, 2.4 G FAT (0.3 G SATURATED), 699.3 MG SODIUM, 1.9 G FIBER, **PE CONTENT 0–5 MG**

8 ounces bean sprouts, stringy ends trimmed
2 cloves garlic, minced
1 teaspoon vegetable oil
2 tablespoons Asian fish sauce (nam pla, nuoc manh, or patis)
1 tablespoon sesame seeds, lightly toasted
1 small red bell pepper, finely shredded, as garnish
Cilantro leaves, as garnish

Heat 4 cups water to boiling in medium saucepan. Add bean sprouts and cook for 30 seconds. Drain well.

Sauté garlic in oil in medium saucepan until light brown and fragrant, about 2 minutes; add fish sauce and bean sprouts. Mix well and transfer to serving dish. Sprinkle with sesame seeds. Garnish with bell pepper and cilantro.

Serve with rice.

Serves 4.

Fresh bean sprouts cook very quickly and do not tolerate reheating at all. They are readily available everywhere and also very cheap. Fresh bean sprouts are sprouted from mung beans and are quite easy to grow at home. Bean sprouts are very rich in vitamin C, the B vitamins, and protein, although it is only a second-class protein. Its phytoestrogens are mainly in the form of lignans and coumestrol. Asian fish sauce (the name varies with the country of origin, but all are similar) can be found in the Asian foods section of large supermarkets, as well as in Asian markets, and can also be obtained by mail order.

CHEESY SCALLOPED POTATOES ★

PER SERVING: 194 CALORIES, 3.7 G PROTEIN, 27.7 G CARBOHYDRATE, 7.9 G FAT (1.6 G SATURATED), 363.3 MG SODIUM, 2.3 G FIBER, **PE CONTENT 0–5 MG**

6 medium boiling potatoes, unpeeled, thinly sliced
½ cup chopped onion
½ cup fat-free milk
1½ cups soy milk
3 tablespoons flour
2 tablespoons soy margarine or butter
1 teaspoon salt or seasoned salt
1 teaspoon dried parsley flakes
Pinch of nutmeg
1 cup (4 ounces) shredded reduced-fat Cheddar cheese
Cayenne pepper, to taste
Paprika, mild or hot, to taste

Spray 9 x 13–inch baking dish with cooking spray. Arrange potato slices and onion in dish.

Combine milk, soy milk, flour, margarine, salt, parsley, and nutmeg in small saucepan. Heat to boiling, stirring constantly; stir in cheese. Season to taste with cayenne pepper. Pour sauce over potatoes; sprinkle with paprika.

Bake at 350° F, covered with aluminum foil, for 1 hour. Uncover and bake an additional 15 minutes, or until golden brown.

Serves 8.

Recipe from *It's Soy Easy…to Cook with Soy*. By permission of the Ohio Soybean Council.

★
★ ★

TOFU IN PASTRY BASKETS

PER SERVING: 268 CALORIES, 8.8 G PROTEIN, 51.3 G CARBOHYDRATE, 4.1 G FAT (0.7 G SATURATED), 585.6 MG SODIUM, 4.9 G FIBER, **PE CONTENT 5–10 MG**

12 frozen spring-roll wrappers (5 x 5–inch)
1 teaspoon vegetable oil
1 egg, lightly beaten
Salt and pepper, to taste
2 cups (4 ounces) mung bean sprouts, stringy ends trimmed
½ cup shredded carrot
2 cups thinly sliced lettuce
4 ounces frozen firm tofu, grilled and shredded
2 ounces chopped cooked shrimp (optional)
Chili Dressing (recipe follows)

Preheat oven to 350° F.

Ease spring-roll wrapper into lightly greased muffin tin; put a paper muffin cup inside each sheet, in order to produce a perfectly shaped basket. Bake pastry with paper muffin cup at 350° F until golden brown, about 10 minutes. Remove paper cups and pastry baskets from tin; cool on wire rake. Store the paper cup away for future use.

Heat oil in small skillet over medium heat. Pour in egg, and sprinkle lightly with salt and pepper. Cook over medium heat, making a thin omelet. Cool; shred thinly.

Blanch bean sprouts in boiling water to cover for 20 seconds; drain. Rinse with cold water; drain and pat dry with paper towels. Combine bean sprouts, omelet, carrot, lettuce, tofu (frozen first, then grilled and shredded), and cooked shrimp, if using, in a large bowl; toss well. Spoon into baskets. Drizzle with Chili Dressing.

Serves 4.

CHILI DRESSING

(makes about ½ cup)

2 tablespoons hot water
1 tablespoon honey
¼ cup Thai sweet chili sauce
2 tablespoons lime juice
⅛ teaspoon salt

Whisk all ingredients in small bowl until smooth.

★

FRIED RICE

PER SERVING: 233 CALORIES, 9.0 G PROTEIN, 31.2 G CARBOHYDRATE, 8.6 G FAT (1.2 G SATURATED), 548.6 MG SODIUM, 2.1 G FIBER, **PE CONTENT 0–5 MG**

1 large egg
Pinch of salt
Pinch of pepper
2 tablespoons plus 2 teaspoons vegetable oil (soybean, peanut, or canola), divided

1 tablespoon plus 1 teaspoon minced onion

4 ounces Chinese barbecued pork (char siew), or packaged lean honey-baked ham, cut into ¼-inch cubes (see note below)

1 cup frozen peas, thawed
3 cups cooked long-grain rice
4 tablespoons light soy sauce
1 tablespoon plus 1 teaspoon oyster sauce
1 medium carrot, shredded
3 cooked shrimp, peeled, deveined, diced (optional)
Cilantro leaves, as garnish

Beat egg, salt, and pepper in small bowl. Heat ½ tablespoon oil in wok over medium heat. When the oil is hot, add the beaten egg and spread over bottom of wok as if cooking a thin crêpe. As soon as egg is cooked, remove from pan—do not overcook, as this will make it rubbery. Cool; cut into ½-inch strips. Reserve.

Heat remaining 2 tablespoons plus ½ teaspoon oil in wok over medium heat. Add onion and stir-fry until fragrant and just starting to brown. Add pork (see note) and peas, and stir-fry 1 minute. Stir in rice, soy sauce, and oyster sauce.

Cook 5 minutes; make a hollow in middle of rice. Add carrot and shrimp (if using); stir-fry 5 minutes longer. Stir in reserved egg. Garnish with cilantro.

Serves 6.

Note: This recipe is easily adapted for low-fat and vegetarian diets. Instead of the barbecued pork you can substitute 1¾ ounces of diced light ham; vegetarians can use 3½ ounces of tofu cutlet, diced into small cubes, or smoked soy "meat."

Main Courses

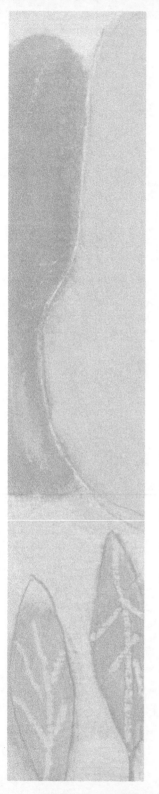

GADO GADO

★
★
★

PER SERVING: 232 CALORIES, 11.3 G PROTEIN, 27.6 G CARBOHYDRATE, 10.7 G FAT
(1.5 G SATURATED), 323.1 MG SODIUM, 5.7 G FIBER, **PE CONTENT 10–15 MG**

½ tablespoon vegetable oil (soybean, peanut, or canola)
10 ounces firm tofu, cut into cubes
3 ½ ounces tempeh, sliced
1 ½ cups green beans, trimmed
4 cups (8 ounces) mung bean sprouts, stringy ends trimmed
1 ½ cup julienne jicama
1 can (11 ounces) pineapple chunks, drained
2 medium tomatoes, cubed
2 cucumbers, cubed
Gado Gado Sauce (recipe follows)

Heat oil in large nonstick skillet over medium heat until hot. Fry tofu and tempeh until brown and crispy. Drain on paper towels.

Drop green beans into boiling salted water to cover. Blanch until crisp-tender (2–3 minutes, depending on thickness). Drain and rinse with cold water until cool; drain well.

Blanch bean sprouts in boiling water to cover for 1 minute; drain well.

Arrange tofu, tempeh, green beans, bean sprouts, jicama, pineapple, tomatoes, and cucumbers on large serving platter. Serve cold with Gado Gado Sauce. Each person selects from the platter and then pours some sauce over their food.

Serves 8.

Gado Gado Sauce

(makes about ¾ cup)

2 tablespoons plus 2 teaspoons hot water
4 tablespoons ketjap manis (see Glossary of Ingredients, page 81)
2 teaspoons minced garlic
2 tablespoons plus 2 teaspoons Asian chili sauce
(see Glossary of Ingredients, page 80)
4 tablespoons (2 ounces) finely chopped roasted peanuts

Combine all ingredients in small bowl.

This dish goes well with coconut-flavored rice and fish, or with plain rice and curries. Green beans contain phytoestrogens. The peanuts, tempeh, and tofu are the main sources of fat in this dish. However, only a small portion of the fat is saturated.

HOT POT (STEAMBOAT)

★
★
★
★
★

Steamboat, the Australian name for Mongolian Hot Pot, is particularly good in cold weather, or whenever you want to linger over a meal, chatting with your fellow diners between courses, watching the dishes cook before your very eyes at the table. Diners cook vegetables, meat, and seafood in broth at the table, adding various sauces to their food, and then they drink the soup remaining in the cooker.

A hot pot is not hard to set up. A Mongolian cooker on charcoal is traditionally placed at the center of the table, with insulation adequate to prevent damage to the table. If you do not have a Mongolian hot pot, a fondue pot, electric rice cooker, or electric wok will do just fine. Meats and vegetables are cooked in stock, and special wire-mesh nets are used to fish the items out. These nets are inexpensive and easily obtained from most Asian grocery stores and from cookware stores and catalogs such as Williams Sonoma and Sur La Table.

Seafood cooks quite quickly in boiling stock, while meats such as pork and chicken take longer. Slicing meats thinly will ensure shorter cooking times. Tofu and all the vegetables listed in this recipe cook very quickly. The bean thread noodles will take about twice as long as the vegetables to cook.

The sauces are placed around the table within easy reach of the diners; recipes will indicate that some sauces go better with certain meats or vegetables.

A suggested amount of different meats and seafoods is given. You can vary the amount of meat and seafood you wish to serve. Cut back on meat if you are on a low animal protein diet.

½ pound shrimp or prawns, peeled, deveined
6 ounces scallops
Salt, to taste
6 ounces boneless lean pork, very thinly sliced
6 ounces boneless lean beef, very thinly sliced
6 ounces boneless, skinless chicken breast, very thinly sliced
6 ounces cleaned squid, cut into bite-size pieces
Cilantro leaves, as garnish
3½ ounces bean thread noodles, soaked in cold water, drained
¾ cup sliced Chinese (Napa) cabbage
1 bunch Chinese chrysanthemum vegetable (watercress is a suitable substitute), well washed
1 bunch green onions, cut into 1½-inch lengths
4 cups (8 ounces) bean sprouts, stringy ends trimmed
1¼ pounds tofu, cubed
3–4 quarts Asian-Style Chicken Stock (see page 88) or canned reduced-sodium chicken broth

Sprinkle shrimp and scallops very lightly with salt. Arrange seafood and meat on large platter and garnish with cilantro. Refrigerate, covered, until ready to use. Arrange noodles, vegetables, and tofu on another large platter. Place on the table with the meat and seafood platter.

Pour 2–3 quarts of stock into the cooker and heat to boiling. Cook items one group at a time to ensure complete and even cooking. For example, beef cooks faster than pork, and bean sprouts cook faster than Chinese cabbage. Use wire-mesh nets to remove the cooked items from the stock.

Eat while hot, dipping individual items into any of the sauces listed on the following pages. Add more stock to the "steamboat" as needed.

Serves 8.

Fragrant Soy Sauce: All of the meats and vegetables listed go very well with this sauce.

Sauté 1 tablespoon diced onion and 1 tablespoon diced garlic in 1 tablespoon soybean oil in small skillet until golden brown. Add a pinch of sugar, 3 tablespoons hot water, and ⅓ cup light soy sauce.

Oyster sauce: Meat, scallops, Chinese cabbage, tofu, Chinese chrysanthemums, and bean sprouts go well with oyster sauce.

Combine 2 teaspoons sesame oil and 2 tablespoons good-quality oyster sauce in small bowl; stir in 1 tablespoon hot water.

Lime and Fish Sauce: Seafood and chicken are excellent with this sauce.

Thinly slice 3 to 4 young lime leaves and 1 red chili pepper. Combine with 3 tablespoons fish sauce, 2 tablespoons lime juice, 1 teaspoon sugar, and 3 tablespoons hot water in small bowl.

Plum Sauce: All meats, as well as some fish, taste good with this sauce.

Mix 1 tablespoon plum sauce with 1 tablespoon hot water and ¼ teaspoon salt in small bowl.

Hoisin Sauce: This sauce goes very well with tofu, beef, squid, and pork.

Mix 1 tablespoon hoisin sauce with 5 teaspoons hot water and 1 teaspoon sesame oil in small bowl.

Tom Yum Sauce: This hot and tangy sauce goes well with any of the meats, seafood, and vegetables, if you do not mind the sauce's heat.

Mix 1 tablespoon tom yum paste with 2 tablespoons hot water, 2 teaspoons lime juice, ¼ teaspoon salt, and 1 teaspoon sugar in small bowl.

Asian Chili Sauce: This sauce goes well with any meat or seafood. Bean sprouts can be eaten with chili sauce if you like your food hot.

Combine ½ cup minced hot chili peppers, 2 cloves minced garlic, 1 teaspoon chopped fresh ginger, 1 teaspoon sugar, and ¾ teaspoon salt with 2–2½ tablespoons white vinegar. Alternatively, use one of the commercial brands of ready-made Asian chili sauce.

Satay Peanut Sauce: All meats and vegetables go with this sauce. Squid, beef, chicken, bean sprouts, tofu, and shrimp taste exceptionally delicious with this sauce.

Sauté 1 tablespoon diced garlic and 1 tablespoon diced onion in 1 tablespoon oil in small saucepan. Add 2 teaspoons curry powder mixed with 2 tablespoons chicken broth. Add 2 finely chopped macadamia nuts and, if available, 6 curry leaves. Sauté until fragrant, and then add 1¼ cups canned unsweetened coconut milk, ½ teaspoon lime juice, and ½ teaspoon sugar. Heat to boiling; remove from heat and add ½ cup finely chopped roasted peanuts.

> You will notice that we've given no calculation of the nutritional content of this recipe. Because this is a versatile dish (you can use any combination of vegetables, meats, sauces, and seafoods), it is impossible to calculate values for the mixture of ingredients that you will use. In practical terms, the meats and vegetables and other items used in this recipe don't fit standard serving sizes anyway. You simply select what you like in the amount that you like, with whatever sauces you like.

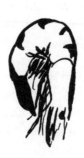

POACHED SPICED CHICKEN ★

PER SERVING: 278 CALORIES, 36.2 G PROTEIN, 19.4 G CARBOHYDRATE, 5.1 G FAT (1.2 G SATURATED),
6,371.5 MG SODIUM, 1.0 G FIBER, **PE CONTENT 0–5 MG**

4 cups water
1 cup light soy sauce
1 cup dark soy sauce
1 tablespoon sugar
2 cloves garlic
2 pieces licorice root (see note below)
1 stick cinnamon
1 star anise (see note below)
10 black peppercorns
1 tablespoon plus 1 teaspoon oyster sauce
*1 tablespoon plus 1 teaspoon Chinese rice wine (Shao Hsing Chiew), dry
sherry, or white wine*
¾-inch piece gingerroot
4 chicken leg/thigh quarters, fat trimmed
Sliced cucumber, sliced tomatoes, fresh cilantro, as garnish

Heat all ingredients, except chicken and garnishes, to boiling in
medium saucepan. Reduce heat and simmer, covered, 5 minutes.

Add chicken to boiling stock. Heat to boiling; turn off heat and let
stand, covered, 15 minutes. Turn chicken pieces over and again heat to
boiling; turn off heat and let stand, covered, 15 minutes, or until juices
run clear when tested with fork.

Garnish with sliced cucumber, tomatoes, and cilantro.

Serve with potatoes or steamed rice.

Serves 4.

Notes: If you can't find star anise and licorice root, use a teaspoon
of Chinese five-spice powder, found in the spice section of large supermarkets, and easily available from mail-order spice catalogs.

The stock can be made ahead of time and frozen until you are
ready to use it. Simply thaw it and continue with the recipe as above.

Beef can be used instead of chicken. You can also use other chicken parts, such as wings, thighs, or breast fillets, but the nutritional information will differ from that given above.

Licorice has very potent antiflushing effects. It can be used in infusion as a beverage. The root is quite sweet and is sold sliced in plastic bags. It may be found in Asian markets and herbal pharmacies, and is available by mail order. People suffering from high blood pressure should not use licorice.

SPICED ROAST CHICKEN ★

PER SERVING: 189 CALORIES, 28.6 G PROTEIN, 6.2 G CARBOHYDRATE, 5.0 G FAT (1.2 G SATURATED),
764.5 MG SODIUM, 1.0 G FIBER, **PE CONTENT 0–5 MG**

2 chicken leg/thigh quarters, fat trimmed
2 tablespoons plus 2 teaspoons light soy sauce
½ teaspoon dried sage leaves
1 teaspoon ground fennel seeds
½ teaspoon ground cinnamon
¼ teaspoon ground star anise
¼ teaspoon pepper
½ teaspoon sugar
2 cloves garlic, finely chopped

Combine chicken and remaining ingredients in glass bowl; turn to coat well. Marinate in refrigerator, covered, at least 4 hours, preferably overnight, turning the chicken pieces occasionally to coat evenly.

Place chicken on rack in roasting pan and roast at 325° F for 40 minutes. Baste with remaining marinade several times during roasting time. Check doneness by puncturing the thigh; if juices run clear with no pink tinge, chicken is ready. Chicken may also be broiled or barbecued.

Serve hot with vegetables and noodles.

Serves 2.

Sage, fennel, and cinnamon all contain phytoestrogens. Soy sauce is made from fermented soybeans and contains very small quantities of phytoestrogens. The oil and fat in this dish drain off during cooking if the chicken is roasted on a rack. If you wish to reduce the fat content of this dish even further, remove the chicken skin before marinating.

★

TERIYAKI CHICKEN

PER SERVING: 167 CALORIES, 20.9 G PROTEIN, 4.1 G CARBOHYDRATE, 7.1 G FAT (1.4 G SATURATED), 987.3 MG SODIUM, 0.0 G FIBER, **PE CONTENT 0–5 MG**

14 ounces chicken thigh, skinned, boned, fat removed
(or chicken breast or fish fillet)
¼ teaspoon sugar
Pinch of salt
⅓ cup teriyaki sauce
1 tablespoon sesame oil, for basting
Lettuce leaves, as garnish

Slice chicken into ¾-inch-thick strips and place in glass baking dish. Sprinkle with sugar and salt. Pour teriyaki sauce over and let marinate, covered, in refrigerator at least 30 minutes.

Cook under a broiler or grill, until juices run clear, about 5 minutes per side, basting with sesame oil and remaining marinade while cooking.

Serve hot on lettuce leaves with plain boiled rice.

Serves 4.

Note: This dish goes very well with rice and stir-fried or steamed vegetables. Other accompaniments, such as raw vegetable salads or pickled radish, ginger, and carrots, can be served with it, too.

Skinned, boned chicken breast can be used instead of thigh; it has much less fat. Fish fillets can be used in place of chicken. In either case, these take less cooking time than chicken thigh, so check each side after 2 minutes and take care not to overcook. When the meat feels springy to the touch, it is done. Teriyaki sauce is made from soybeans and also contains wine, wheat, and spices.

SESAME CHICKEN   ★

PER SERVING: 189 CALORIES, 27.9 G PROTEIN, 3.3 G CARBOHYDRATE, 6.1 G FAT (1.0 G SATURATED), 441.7 MG SODIUM, 0.7 G FIBER, **PE CONTENT 0–5 MG**

1 pound chicken breast fillet, cubed
1 tablespoon plus 1 teaspoon Chinese rice wine or dry sherry
1 tablespoon light soy sauce
1 tablespoon oyster sauce
1 clove garlic, minced
2 teaspoons tahini (see Glossary of Ingredients, page 82)
1 teaspoon sesame oil
1¼-inch piece gingerroot, thinly sliced
2 tablespoons sesame seeds
¼ teaspoon salt

Combine chicken, wine, soy sauce, salt, oyster sauce, garlic, and tahini in glass bowl; marinate in refrigerator, covered, 1 hour.

Heat sesame oil in wok over medium heat until hot; stir-fry ginger until fragrant, about 2 minutes. Increase heat to medium-high; add chicken and stir-fry until well browned, about 8 minutes. Stir in sesame seeds and cook 1 minute.

Serve with steamed vegetables and rice.

Serves 4.

Note: Although the last four chicken dishes are higher in fat content than other dishes in this recipe book, removing all visible fats and skins and draining away the oil will help reduce the overall fat content. These recipes demonstrate how you can turn a neutral meat into an estrogenic dish to your advantage by incorporating estrogenic herbs and spices in the recipes.

This dish is traditionally cooked for new mothers using much more ginger. The dish's nutritional and estrogen content helps to buffer a woman from the rapid plunge in natural estrogen levels that follows the birth of a baby. Phytoestrogens are present in whole sesame seeds, sesame oil, and tahini. Fresh ginger contains a natural anticoagulant that helps prevent deep venous thrombosis and pulmonary embolism (clots in the legs and lungs).

★
★
★

CHICKEN BREASTS WITH
CHIPOTLE SAUCE

PER SERVING: 248 CALORIES, 20.4 G PROTEIN, 15.0 G CARBOHYDRATE, 9.0 G FAT (1.6 G SATURATED), 255.6 MG SODIUM, 3.4 G FIBER, **PE CONTENT 10–15 MG**

4 skinless chicken-breast halves
3 cups Asian-Style Chicken Stock (see page 88) or canned
reduced-sodium chicken broth
1 small onion
1 small carrot
1 small rib celery with leaves
6 whole black peppercorns
Chipotle Sauce (recipe follows)
3 tomatoes, peeled, diced, as garnish
1 green onion, finely chopped

Combine chicken, stock, onion, carrot, celery, and peppercorns in large saucepan; heat to boiling. Skim gray foam from surface and immediately remove pan from heat, cover, and let stand until the chicken is springy to the touch, about 15 minutes.

Drain chicken breasts, reserving stock for another use. Place chicken on serving plates and spoon Chipotle Sauce over it. (For a dressier presentation, lift meat carefully off the bone, slice, and arrange in a fan on each plate.) Sprinkle with tomatoes and green onion.

This very spicy dish calls for rice and warmed tortillas to accompany it, along with a vegetable or salad.

Serves 4.

CHIPOTLE SAUCE

(makes about 2 cups)

*¾ cup Asian-Style Chicken Stock (see page 88), or canned
reduced-sodium chicken broth*
¾ cup mashed silken tofu
¼ cup minced onion
*1 to 2 tablespoons canned chipotle chiles in adobo sauce,
sauce scraped off, seeded*
3 tablespoons peanut butter
Salt, to taste

Process all ingredients, except salt, in food processor or blender
until smooth. Pour into medium saucepan and heat to simmering. Stir
over low heat for 5 minutes. Strain sauce into small bowl, pressing on
sieve with back of spoon. If sauce is too thick, stir in additional stock;
season to taste with salt.

Recipe from Naomi Wise.

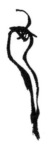

★
★
★
★
★

TACOS

PER SERVING: 355 CALORIES, 14.6 G PROTEIN, 35.2 G CARBOHYDRATE, 18.4 G FAT
(4.3 G SATURATED), 511.1 MG SODIUM, 6.9 G FIBER, **PE CONTENT 20–25 MG**

1 pound firm tofu, crumbled
2 tablespoons vegetable oil (soybean, peanut, canola)
1 package (1.25 ounces) taco seasoning
½ cup water
6 corn tortillas, warmed
1 can (15 ounces) refried beans, heated
Chopped tomatoes, sliced lettuce, sliced green onions, as garnish
Salsa, as garnish

Sauté tofu in oil in large skillet until browned, about 10 minutes. Add taco seasoning and water. Cook until the sauce is thick, about 5 minutes.

To serve, spread tortillas with refried beans and top with tofu. Sprinkle with garnishes; top with salsa and roll up.

Serves 6.

Recipe courtesy of the Indiana Soybean Board.

FESTIVE VEGETABLE FAJITA WRAPS

★
★
★
★
★
★
+

PER SERVING: 258 CALORIES, 20.6 G PROTEIN, 26.8 G CARBOHYDRATE, 9.2 G FAT (2.2 G SATURATED), 195.6 MG SODIUM, 5.0 G FIBER, **PE CONTENT OVER 25 MG**

1 ½ cups cooked soybeans (see page 87)
½ cup chopped red onion
½ cup chopped green bell pepper
½ cup chopped yellow, red, or orange bell pepper
1 jalapeño or serrano chile, seeded, chopped
1 chipotle chile, chopped
2 tablespoons lime juice
2 tablespoons chopped cilantro
½ teaspoon chopped garlic
¼ teaspoon ground cumin seeds
½ cup (2 ounces) shredded reduced-fat Cheddar cheese
8 soft corn or flour tortillas
1 cup bean sprouts
Salsa, guacamole, low-fat sour cream, as garnishes

Preheat oven to 350° F

Combine all ingredients, except tortillas, bean sprouts, and garnishes, in large bowl; mix well. Spoon filling across center of tortillas and top with bean sprouts. Roll up.

Place tortillas, seam down, in 9 x 13–inch baking dish. Bake uncovered at 350° F until vegetables are warm and cheese is melted, about 10 minutes. Serve fajitas with garnishes.

Serves 4.

Note: For a different twist, add 1 cup sliced grilled chicken or beef and 1 cup shredded Monterey Jack cheese to the filling.

Recipe from *It's Soy Easy…to Cook with Soy.* By permission of the Ohio Soybean Council.

★
★
★

HEALTHY CHILI

PER SERVING: 582 CALORIES, 24.9 G PROTEIN, 92.0 G CARBOHYDRATE, 15.4 G FAT (2.2 G SATURATED), 1,139.3 MG SODIUM, 14.2 G FIBER, **PE CONTENT 10–15 MG**

2 cups crumbled firm tofu
1 clove garlic, minced
1 tablespoon chili powder
2 tablespoons Worcestershire sauce
1 cup chopped onion
1 large green pepper, chopped
1 carrot, thinly sliced
2 tablespoons vegetable oil
1 cup chopped seeded tomatoes
1 can (16 ounces) tomato sauce

1 can (15 ounces) dark red kidney beans
1 teaspoon dried basil leaves, crushed
1 teaspoon ground cumin seeds
1 teaspoon cayenne pepper
6 ounces tomato paste (optional)
Salt, to taste
4 cups cooked brown or white rice, warm
Chopped onion, grated Cheddar cheese, avocado, as garnish

Combine tofu, garlic, chili powder, and Worcestershire sauce in small bowl; set aside.

Sauté onion, green pepper, and carrot in oil in large skillet until onion is tender, about 5 minutes. Add tofu mixture and cook 3 minutes over medium heat. Add tomatoes, tomato sauce, kidney beans, basil, cumin, cayenne, and, if desired, tomato paste. Heat to boiling; reduce heat and simmer, covered, 30 minutes. Season to taste with salt. Serve over rice, and sprinkle with garnishes.

Serves 8.

Note: If there is time, refrigerate overnight to blend flavors, then reheat gently.

Recipe used courtesy of the Indiana Soybean Board.

CURRIED TOFU AND VEGETABLES ★★

PER SERVING: 101 CALORIES, 4.8 G PROTEIN, 10.9 G CARBOHYDRATE, 5.1 G FAT (0.7 G SATURATED), 293.1 MG SODIUM, 2.8 G FIBER, **PE CONTENT 5–10 MG**

¼ cup chopped onion
¾-inch piece gingerroot, chopped
1 tablespoon vegetable oil (soybean, canola, olive)
1 tablespoon plus 1 teaspoon curry powder
1¼ cup vegetable broth, divided
10 ounces uncooked pumpkin or winter squash, peeled, cut into 1-inch cubes
1½ cups cut green beans (1-inch)
7 ounces baked hard tofu
1 eggplant, preferably Asian eggplant (7–10 ounces), cut into 1-inch cubes
2 macadamia nuts, ground (or 6 cashews or almonds)
½ teaspoon salt

Sauté onion and ginger in oil in medium saucepan for 2 minutes. Combine curry powder with ¼ cup broth in small bowl to make a paste. Add to onion mixture, and sauté 2–3 minutes, or until very fragrant.

Add pumpkin, and sauté until lightly browned, about 5 minutes. Stir in remaining 1 cup broth and remaining ingredients, except salt. Heat to boiling; reduce heat and simmer, covered, until vegetables are tender, about 20 minutes. Season to taste with salt.

Serve hot with rice, bread, or noodles.

Serves 6.

Note: Fresh shelled and deveined shrimp can be added 8 to 10 minutes before the end of the cooking time, if desired.

> The best result with this recipe is obtained with deep-fried tofu, but the fat content is a drawback. Hence, we have listed baked hard/firm tofu here. Deep-fried tofu has twice the PE content found in firm tofu. If the former is used here, then the PE content for each serving would be 15–20 MG.

★
★
★
★
★

VEGETABLE TOFU STIR-FRY

PER SERVING: 148 CALORIES, 10.2 G PROTEIN, 11.1 G CARBOHYDRATE, 8.5 G FAT (1.2 G SATURATED), 715.4 MG SODIUM, 3.8 G FIBER, **PE CONTENT 20–25 MG**

1 teaspoon minced gingerroot
1 clove garlic, minced
1 tablespoon vegetable oil
14 ounces extra-firm tofu, cut into ¾-inch cubes
1 cup broccoli florets
1 small red bell pepper, diced
1 large carrot, grated
¼ cup sliced water chestnuts
1 tablespoon light soy sauce
1 tablespoon oyster sauce
1 teaspoon salt
⅛ teaspoon pepper

Sauté ginger and garlic in oil in large skillet 1 minute. Add tofu and sauté until lightly browned, 3 to 5 minutes.

Add broccoli, bell pepper, carrot, and water chestnuts; sauté until crisp-tender, about 4 minutes. Add soy sauce, oyster sauce, salt, and pepper; gently stir to heat.

Serve over rice.

Serves 4.

Recipe from *Delicious and Easy Recipes for Tofu and Pasta*. By permission of Azumaya.

Tofu in Oyster Sauce

★
★
★
★
★

PER SERVING: 93 CALORIES, 5.2 G PROTEIN, 5.9 G CARBOHYDRATE, 5.1 G FAT (0.5 G SATURATED), 369.4 MG SODIUM, 0.5 G FIBER, **PE CONTENT 20–25 MG**

1 tablespoon soybean oil, divided
10 ounces silken tofu, cut into 6 pieces
1 clove garlic, diced
1 small red onion, diced
2 tablespoons oyster sauce
1 tablespoon light soy sauce
¼ cup Asian-Style Chicken Stock (see page 88)
or canned reduced-sodium chicken or vegetable broth
½ teaspoon cornstarch
Ground black pepper, to taste
Cilantro or celery leaves, as garnish

Heat ½ tablespoon oil in wok over medium–high heat. Stir-fry tofu over medium–high heat until golden brown; be gentle as it breaks very easily. Transfer to serving dish.

Stir-fry garlic and onion in wok in remaining ½ tablespoon oil until fragrant, about 3 minutes. Reduce heat to low. Add combined oyster sauce, soy sauce, stock, and cornstarch. Heat to boiling, stirring constantly; season to taste with pepper. Pour over tofu. Garnish with cilantro.

Serve hot, accompanied by steamed rice and stir-fried vegetable dishes.

Serves 4.

★
★
★
★
★

TOFU WITH GROUND MEAT

PER SERVING: 139 CALORIES, 9.5 G PROTEIN, 8.8 G CARBOHYDRATE, 6.6 G FAT (1.6 G SATURATED),
681.9 MG SODIUM, 0.1 G FIBER, **PE CONTENT 20–25 MG**

3 ½ ounces lean ground meat (chicken breast, pork, beef, lamb, or turkey)
1 tablespoon plus 1 teaspoon light soy sauce
1 tablespoon plus 1 teaspoon oyster sauce
1 teaspoon Chinese rice wine or dry sherry
2 tablespoons plus 2 teaspoons cornstarch, divided
1 clove garlic, minced
1 teaspoon vegetable oil
10 ounces silken tofu, cut into ½-inch cubes
1 tablespoon plus 1 teaspoon dark soy sauce
¼ teaspoon sugar
¼ cup water
Salt and pepper, to taste
Cilantro leaves or sliced green onion, as garnish

Combine meat, light soy sauce, oyster sauce, wine, and 1 tablespoon plus 1 teaspoon cornstarch in small bowl. Let stand 10 minutes.

Sauté garlic in oil in wok or large skillet until fragrant, about 1 minute. Add meat mixture and cook over high heat until lightly browned, about 5 minutes. Add tofu and dark soy sauce. Cook, covered, over medium heat 2–3 minutes.

Combine remaining 1 tablespoon plus 1 teaspoon cornstarch, sugar, and water in small bowl; add to wok. Heat to boiling, stirring until thickened, about 1 minute. Season to taste with salt and pepper. Spoon into serving bowl; garnish with cilantro.

Serve over rice.

Serves 4.

This is a popular Cantonese dish that is easy to prepare and cook. Ground pork is normally used, but julienne-cut beef or chicken breast fillets can be substituted, resulting in different flavors. Pork is much higher in fat than chicken breast fillets. Use the latter for a lower fat version. An accompanying dish such as steamed vegetables or a stir-fried combination is most suitable.

★
★
★
★
★
+

HUNANESE TOFU BEEF

PER SERVING: 323 CALORIES, 20.1 G PROTEIN, 8.9 G CARBOHYDRATE, 22.7 G FAT (4.5 G SATURATED),
514.1 MG SODIUM, 0.9 G FIBER, **PE CONTENT OVER 25 MG**

1 pound firm tofu, cubed (½-inch), dried on paper towels
4 large garlic cloves, minced
1 large green onion, chopped
1 tablespoon chopped gingerroot
3 tablespoons vegetable oil
½ cup finely chopped carrots or green beans
6 ounces lean ground beef
½ cup Asian-Style Chicken Stock (see page 88), or canned
reduced-sodium chicken broth
2 tablespoons light soy sauce
1 tablespoon Chinese rice wine (Shao Hsing) or dry sherry
1 tablespoon Asian chili sauce
¼ teaspoon sugar
¼ teaspoon salt
1½ teaspoons cornstarch
1½ tablespoons water
Ground black pepper, to taste

Fry tofu as directed for deep-fried tofu (see page 90).

Stir-fry garlic, green onion, and ginger in oil in wok over medium-high heat about 30 seconds (do not brown). Add carrots or green beans and cook 1 minute. Add ground beef and stir-fry over medium-high heat until meat browns, crumbling meat with chopsticks or wooden spoon. Stir in stock, soy sauce, rice wine, and chili sauce. Gently stir in tofu and heat to simmering. Stir in combined sugar, salt, cornstarch, and water; simmer until sauce thickens slightly. Season to taste with pepper.

Serve over rice, if desired.

Serves 4.

Recipe from Naomi Wise.

STEAMED FISH WITH TOFU

★
★
★
★
★

PER SERVING: 121 CALORIES, 14.0 G PROTEIN, 4.2 G CARBOHYDRATE, 5.0 G FAT (0.7 G SATURATED), 194.6 MG SODIUM, 0.1 G FIBER, **PE CONTENT 20–25 MG**

*7 ounces firm boneless white fish fillet, such as lingcod, rock cod,
or sea bass, cut into ½-inch strips*
1 tablespoon oyster sauce
1 tablespoon soy sauce
1 teaspoon Chinese rice wine (Shao Hsing) or dry sherry
12 thin slices gingerroot
1 tablespoon plus 1 teaspoon cornstarch
½ tablespoon vegetable oil (soybean, peanut, canola)
1 clove garlic, minced
10 ounces low fat silken firm tofu, cut into sheets ½-inch thick
Sliced green onion or cilantro, as garnish

Combine fish, oyster sauce, soy sauce, wine, ginger, and cornstarch in glass bowl; toss to coat well. Refrigerate, covered, 20–30 minutes.

Sauté garlic in oil in small skillet until light brown. Brush ceramic or glass baking dish with ½ the garlic oil, and arrange tofu in dish.

Place portions of the fish on each tofu piece. Brush top of fish with remaining garlic oil and top with ginger slices.

Pour about ½ inch of water into the bottom of a steamer, or a covered roaster with rack. Place the dish in steamer or on rack. Cover; heat water to boiling, and steam 10 minutes, or until fish flakes with a fork. Sprinkle with green onion.

Serve hot with steamed rice.

Serves 4.

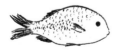

Whole fish, such as snapper, rock cod, or black cod, can be steamed with tofu, but score the sides of the fish before marinating. Make sure your tofu is fresh; otherwise the dish will turn sour in taste.

★
★
★
★
★

SWEET AND SOUR TOFU

PER SERVING: 137 CALORIES, 5.3 G PROTEIN, 13.4 G CARBOHYDRATE, 7.6 G FAT (1.0 G SATURATED), 416.4 MG SODIUM, 1.6 G FIBER, **PE CONTENT 20–25 MG**

2 tablespoons oil, divided
10 ounces low-fat silken firm tofu, cut into ¾-inch cubes
½ medium carrot, julienned
2 tablespoons plus 2 teaspoons apple cider vinegar
1 medium onion
½ teaspoon salt
2 tablespoons plus 2 teaspoons tomato sauce or ketchup
¾ cup cucumber chunks
½ cup pineapple chunks
½ medium red bell pepper, cubed
1 tablespoon plus 1 teaspoon sugar
½ teaspoon cornstarch
2 tablespoons water
Ground black pepper, to taste

Heat 1 tablespoon oil in wok over high heat; fry tofu until golden brown, turning gently to brown all sides. Remove from wok and reserve.

Combine carrot and vinegar in small bowl. Cut onion into 8 wedges; separate each wedge into segments. Sauté onion in remaining 1 tablespoon oil in wok for 2 minutes; add carrot mixture and cook 1 minute. Stir in salt, tomato sauce, cucumber, pineapple, bell pepper, sugar, and combined cornstarch and water. Heat to boiling and add tofu, stirring gently until heated through. Season to taste with pepper.

Serve hot with steamed rice.

Serves 4.

Note: Tempeh can be used instead of tofu in this recipe. Tempeh is rather salty and stronger in flavor than tofu, so use only 5 ounces. Cut into smaller cubes and fry until brown before adding to the sweet and sour mixture.

TOFU AND MUSHROOM PARCELS

★
★
★
★

PER SERVING: 211 CALORIES, 9.4 G PROTEIN, 26.8 G CARBOHYDRATE, 7.2 G FAT (1.2 G SATURATED),
412.5 MG SODIUM, 2.5 G FIBER, **PE CONTENT 15–20 MG**

4 ounces mushrooms, chopped
1 medium onion, chopped
¾ cup chopped parsley
7 ounces tofu cutlet (see page 92), diced
1 teaspoon chicken or vegetable bouillon crystals
1 tablespoon medium sherry or white wine
Pinch of ground black pepper
8 sheets fillo pastry, thawed
Vegetable cooking spray
2 tablespoons sesame seeds

Preheat oven to 325° F.

Combine mushrooms, onion, parsley, tofu, bouillon, sherry, and pepper in large bowl.

Stack 4 sheets fillo on counter, spraying each lightly with cooking spray. Spoon half of the mushroom mixture in center of fillo. Fold fillo over filling in thirds, like you're folding a letter; turn over and place on lightly greased baking sheet so that free edge is underneath, tucking both ends under. Repeat with remaining fillo and filling. Spray generously with vegetable oil and sprinkle with sesame seeds.

Bake at 325° F until golden brown, about 30 minutes.

Serves 4.

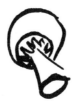

★ Stir-Fried Baby Bok Choy and Tofu
★
★
★

PER SERVING: 113 CALORIES, 8.2 G PROTEIN, 7.1 G CARBOHYDRATE, 6.3 G FAT (0.5 G SATURATED), 728.7 MG SODIUM, 2.4 G FIBER, **PE CONTENT 15–20 MG**

2 cloves garlic, chopped
½ tablespoon vegetable oil (canola, peanut, soybean)
3½ ounces tofu cutlet (see page 92), thinly sliced (⅛ inch thick)
1 bunch (10–12 ounces) baby bok choy, quartered lengthwise
2 teaspoons oyster sauce
2 teaspoons light soy sauce
1 teaspoon cornstarch
¼ cup canned reduced-sodium chicken or vegetable broth

Sauté garlic in oil in large saucepan until fragrant and light brown, about 2 minutes. Add tofu and sauté 1 minute. Add bok choy and sauté 2 minutes. Add oyster and soy sauces and cook, covered, 1 minute. Combine cornstarch and broth. Stir broth mixture into tofu mixture; cook, stirring, until thickened.

Serve hot with rice, noodles, or pasta.

Serves 2.

EIGHT-TREASURED CHAP CHOY

★
★
★

PER SERVING: 184 CALORIES, 7.8 G PROTEIN, 13.5 G CARBOHYDRATE, 11.1 G FAT (1.7 G SATURATED), 350.1 MG SODIUM, 3.8 G FIBER, **PE CONTENT 5–10 MG**

½ cup cubed carrot (½ inch)
½ cup cauliflower florets
2 cloves garlic, chopped
1 tablespoon vegetable oil (canola, peanut, soybean)
½ cup cubed (½ inch) tofu cutlet (see page 92)
1½ tablespoons oyster or stir-fry sauce
1 tablespoon light soy sauce
1 tablespoon medium sherry or white wine
½ cup frozen peas, thawed
4 ounces mushrooms, quartered
½ cup diced red or yellow bell peppers
½ cup diced celery
1 teaspoon cornstarch
¼ cup canned reduced-sodium chicken or vegetable broth
2 ounces cashews

Blanch carrots and cauliflower in boiling water to cover for 2 minutes; drain.

Sauté garlic in oil in wok or large skillet until fragrant, about 1 minute. Add tofu, oyster sauce, soy sauce, sherry, carrots, cauliflower, peas, and mushrooms. Sauté 2 minutes. Stir in peppers and celery and cook, covered, 1 minute.

Mix cornstarch and broth in small bowl; add to wok. Stir until sauce is thickened.

Spoon onto serving plate; sprinkle with cashews.

Serve with rice, noodles, or pasta.

Serves 4.

★
★
★
★

EGGPLANT IN MISO SAUCE

PER SERVING: 225 CALORIES, 8.9 G PROTEIN, 21.0 G CARBOHYDRATE, 10.5 G FAT (2.0 G SATURATED), 324.6 MG SODIUM, 4.5 G FIBER, **PE CONTENT 15–20 MG**

2 ounces ground meat (pork, beef, lamb, chicken, or shrimp)
2 tablespoons low-salt miso paste, divided
2 tablespoons medium sherry or wine
Pinch of pepper
2 medium eggplants (about 1 pound)
1 small onion, chopped
1 clove garlic, chopped
1 tablespoon vegetable oil (canola, peanut, soybean)
3½ ounces tofu cutlet (see page 92), finely diced
1 teaspoon cornstarch
⅓ cup canned reduced-sodium chicken or vegetable broth, divided
Cilantro, as garnish
1 tablespoon finely chopped red chili, as garnish

Combine meat, 1 tablespoon miso paste, wine, and pepper in small bowl; let stand while preparing eggplant.

Cover eggplant with boiling water in deep saucepan. Heat to boiling; simmer, covered, until tender, about 20 minutes. Cool in cold water; peel off skins. Cut lengthwise into quarters.

Sauté onion and garlic in oil in large skillet until light brown, about 3 minutes. Stir in meat mixture and cook until meat is done, about 3 minutes. Stir in remaining 1 tablespoon miso paste and tofu and cook 1 minute. Combine cornstarch and broth in small bowl. Stir into meat mixture; heat to boiling. Stir in eggplant; stir until hot.

Spoon into serving bowl; sprinkle with cilantro and chopped red chili.

Serves 3.

Baked Fish in Miso Sauce

PER SERVING: 303 CALORIES, 32.8 G PROTEIN, 12.1 G CARBOHYDRATE, 9.2 G FAT (1.4 G SATURATED), 508.3 MG SODIUM, 0.1 G FIBER, **PE CONTENT 5–10 MG**

12 ounces lean white fish fillets
3 tablespoons medium sherry or white wine
2 tablespoons low-salt miso paste
2 cloves garlic, minced
2 teaspoons finely chopped gingerroot
Lime juice, to taste

Preheat oven to 325° F.

Place fish on large piece of aluminum foil. Mix wine, miso paste, garlic, and gingerroot in small bowl; pour over fish, turning to coat both sides. Bring edges of foil together, sealing carefully. Place packet on baking sheet. Bake at 325° F until packet puffs and fish flakes when tested with a fork, about 20 minutes. Open packet; sprinkle with lime juice.

Serve hot with steamed vegetables, rice, or noodles.

Serves 2.

★
★
★
★
★
+

Corn Bread Tamale Pie

PER SERVING: 379 CALORIES, 15.4 G PROTEIN, 58.9 G CARBOHYDRATE, 11.1 G FAT (1.9 G
SATURATED), 1,379.4 MG SODIUM, 9.6 G FIBER, **PE CONTENT 20–25 MG**

Vegetable cooking spray
1 medium onion, chopped
2–3 cloves garlic, minced
½ cup chopped green bell pepper
½ cup chopped red bell pepper
2 medium zucchini, cut into ½-inch cubes
1 medium eggplant, cubed
10 ounces firm tofu, drained, crumbled
10–12 mushrooms, sliced
1 cup tomato sauce or puree
1 cup canned reduced-sodium chicken or vegetable broth
¼ teaspoon pepper
1 teaspoon salt
1 tablespoon chili powder
Pinch of cayenne pepper
1 cup whole-kernel corn
Tamale Topping (recipe follows)

Spray large skillet with cooking spray; heat over medium heat until
hot. Sauté onion, garlic, bell peppers, zucchini, eggplant, tofu, and
mushrooms until tofu is lightly browned and onion is translucent,
about 10 minutes. Add remaining ingredients, except Tamale Topping.
Heat to boiling; reduce heat and simmer, uncovered, until slightly
thickened, about 5 minutes.

Place vegetable mixture into lightly greased 11 x 7–inch baking
dish and spoon Tamale Topping over it. (Note: Topping may sink to the
bottom, but will rise when baked.) Bake at 400° F until topping is
nicely browned, about 20–25 minutes.

Serves 4–6.

TAMALE TOPPING

¾ cup yellow cornmeal
1 tablespoon flour
1 tablespoon sugar
½ teaspoon salt
1½ teaspoons baking powder
1 egg, lightly beaten
⅓ cup soy milk
1 tablespoon vegetable oil
1 teaspoon finely chopped jalapeño chile

Mix cornmeal, flour, sugar, salt, and baking powder in medium bowl. Beat egg, soy milk, and vegetable oil in small bowl. Stir into flour mixture. Add jalapeño and stir just to combine.

Recipe from *Healthy and Delicious Recipes, Vol. 1.* By permission of VitaSoy.

★
★
★
★
★
+

Stewed Bean Curd Skin and Cloud Ears with Pork

PER SERVING: 170 CALORIES, 14.6 G PROTEIN, 8.4 G CARBOHYDRATE, 8.4 G FAT (1.8 G SATURATED), 537.7 MG SODIUM, 2.6 G FIBER, **PE CONTENT OVER 25 MG**

¾ ounce cloud ears or tree ears (wood fungus or wood mushrooms)
3½ ounces bean curd skin (also called bean curd sticks or bamboo yuba)
7 ounces pork country ribs (from loin) or center-cut pork chops,
fat trimmed, cubed
1 tablespoon plus 1 teaspoon Chinese rice wine (Shao Hsing) or dry sherry
2 tablespoons plus 2 teaspoons dark soy sauce
2 tablespoons plus 2 teaspoons red fermented bean curd (optional)
¼ teaspoon sugar
4 cloves garlic, chopped
1 tablespoon plus 1 teaspoon vegetable oil (soybean, peanut, canola)
1¼ cups water, divided
½ teaspoon cornstarch
Ground black pepper, to taste
Cilantro leaves, as garnish

Soak cloud ears in hot water in small bowl for 30 minutes; remove any debris, and change water if necessary. Break the bean curd skin into 1¾- to 2-inch lengths; soak in hot water in small bowl 30 minutes.

Combine pork, wine, dark soy sauce, fermented bean curd, and sugar in medium bowl. Let stand 10 minutes. (Bones from the meat may be left whole if they can't be cut. Include them in the stew as they contribute flavor and calcium.)

Sauté garlic in oil in large saucepan until fragrant, about 1 minute. Add pork mixture; sauté until browned, about 5 minutes.

Drain cloud ears and bean curd skin, discarding water; if cloud ears are not shredded, cut into small pieces. Add cloud ears and bean curd skin to saucepan. Sauté 5 minutes, then add 1 cup of water. Heat to boiling; reduce heat and simmer, covered, until pork is tender, about 40 minutes.

Mix cornstarch and remaining ¼ cup water in small bowl; stir into stew 5 minutes before end of cooking time. Season to taste with pepper, and garnish with cilantro.

Serve hot with steamed/boiled rice and steamed green vegetables. Serves 6.

The fat content of this dish can be reduced by using lean cubed chicken meat in place of pork.

Wood fungus or wood mushroom is also known as **cloud ear**, **wood ear**, and **tree ear**. An albino form of this mushroom is called **silver ear**. Dehydrated, packaged wood fungus can be bought from Asian food stores and some large supermarkets. It is available shredded or whole, and it has to be soaked in hot water before use. It swells 5 to 6 times in size and resembles an ear after reconstituting; hence the common names. Wood fungus is reputed to possess anticoagulation properties that decrease the stickiness of platelets in the blood.

Bean curd skins, available from Asian groceries and some health-food stores, are known as **bean curd sticks** or **bamboo yuba** in some countries. Protein content varies greatly among the various brands of this product.

Fermented red bean curd (a.k.a. **bean cheese**) is available from Asian groceries. It has a rich, powerful flavor, similar to gorgonzola cheese. Once gotten used to, the flavor can be addictive.

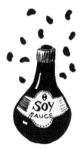

★
★
★
★
★
★

STIR-FRIED TEMPEH AND VEGETABLES

PER SERVING: 255 CALORIES, 15.4 G PROTEIN, 28.9 G CARBOHYDRATE, 10.2 G FAT (1.8 G
SATURATED), 1,503.0 MG SODIUM, 8.871 G FIBER, **PE CONTENT 20–25 MG**

3½ ounces tempeh
2 teaspoons cornstarch, divided
2 cloves garlic, chopped
2 teaspoons vegetable oil (soybean, peanut, or canola)
1 medium carrot, sliced or julienned
1 cup whole baby corn, each ear halved lengthwise
⅓ cup small broccoli florets
¾ cup sugar snap peas, ends trimmed
½ medium red bell pepper, cubed
2 tablespoons plus 1 teaspoon oyster sauce
1 tablespoon plus 1 teaspoon light soy sauce
¼ teaspoon salt
⅓ cup water
Ground black pepper, to taste

Cut tempeh into ¼-inch-thick slices, and then cut each slice into
3 pieces. Sprinkle 1½ teaspoons cornstarch over tempeh in small bowl
and toss to coat.

Sauté garlic in oil in wok or large skillet. Add tempeh and sauté
until brown, about 5 minutes. Add carrot and cook 2 minutes; add
corn and cook 2 minutes. Stir in broccoli, sugar snap peas, bell pepper,
oyster sauce, soy sauce, and salt. Cook 2 minutes. Mix remaining ½ teaspoon cornstarch with water and add to vegetables. Cook, covered,
1 minute; season to taste with pepper.

Serve with steamed rice or noodles.

Serves 2.

STIR-FRIED PRAWNS, SNOW PEAS, AND TOFU

★
★
★
★

PER SERVING: 225 CALORIES, 16.6 G PROTEIN, 15.7 G CARBOHYDRATE, 10.7 G FAT (1.3 G SATURATED), 1,327.8 MG SODIUM, 1.2 G FIBER, **PE CONTENT 15–20 MG**

> *7 ounces prawns or large shrimp, peeled, deveined*
> *2 tablespoons plus 2 teaspoons soy sauce, divided*
> *2 tablespoons oyster sauce, divided*
> *1 teaspoon Chinese rice wine, dry sherry, or dry white wine*
> *10 ounces firm tofu, cubed (1½-inch), dried on paper toweling*
> *4 tablespoons cornstarch, divided*
> *2 tablespoons vegetable oil, divided*
> *1¼ cups snow peas, trimmed*
> *1 medium onion, sliced*
> *¼ cup plus 1 tablespoon chicken stock, divided*
> *½ teaspoon salt*
> *½ teaspoon sugar*

Combine prawns, 1 tablespoon plus 1 teaspoon soy sauce, 1 tablespoon oyster sauce, and wine in medium glass bowl; let stand 10 minutes.

Coat tofu with 2 tablespoons cornstarch. Heat 1 tablespoon cooking oil over high heat in large nonstick skillet or wok; when oil is smoking, fry tofu until browned on all sides. Remove from skillet; drain off excess oil, and arrange tofu on serving plate.

In clean wok or skillet, heat remaining 1 tablespoon oil over medium heat. Stir-fry marinated shrimp until pink and curled, about 3 minutes; remove from wok. Add snow peas and onion, and stir-fry 4 minutes. Add 1 tablespoon stock, the remaining 1 tablespoon of oyster sauce and soy sauce, sugar, and salt. Return shrimp to wok. Mix the remaining 2 tablespoons cornstarch with remaining ¼ cup stock, and add to wok. Stir over high heat until thickened, about 2 minutes.

Spoon shrimp mixture over cooked tofu.

Serve with rice or instant cooked noodles.

Serves 4.

★
★
TOFU CUTLET IN LETTUCE LEAVES WITH PRAWNS

PER SERVING: 98 CALORIES, 5.6 G PROTEIN, 8.8 G CARBOHYDRATE, 5.6 G FAT (0.8 G SATURATED), 154.7 MG SODIUM, 1.1 G FIBER, **PE CONTENT 5–10 MG**

3½ ounces prawns or large shrimp, peeled, deveined
1 teaspoon light soy sauce
¾ ounce dried shiitake mushrooms
2 tablespoons oil (soybean, peanut, canola)
1 medium onion, chopped
1 stalk celery, chopped
⅔ cup chopped water chestnuts
3½ ounces grilled tofu cutlet (see page 91), cut into ¼-inch cubes
1 teaspoon cornstarch
¼ cup water
¼ teaspoon salt
¼ teaspoon pepper
12 lettuce leaves (preferably iceberg), trimmed into rounds

Cut prawns into ¼-inch pieces; combine with light soy sauce in small bowl and let stand 10 minutes. Soak mushrooms in hot water for 10 minutes or until softened; rinse well and chop, discarding tough stems.

Heat oil in wok over high heat until hot. Stir-fry onion 2 minutes; add mushrooms and stir-fry 5 minutes. Stir in celery, water chestnuts, and tofu. Combine cornstarch, water, salt, and pepper in small bowl. Stir into wok; add prawns and continue stirring until prawns are cooked and mixture is almost dry, about 4 minutes.

Spoon mixture into lettuce rounds. Serve immediately.

Serves 6.

This dish can be served as an appetizer, or as an entrée with steamed rice and salads.

SOYBEAN SPROUTS WITH GROUND MEAT

★
★
★
★
★
+

PER SERVING: 80 CALORIES, 4.9 G PROTEIN, 2.3 G CARBOHYDRATE, 5.4 G FAT (0.5 G SATURATED),
479.3 MG SODIUM, 0.1 G FIBER, **PE CONTENT OVER 25 MG**

4 cups (13 ounces) soybean sprouts (see page 51–52 for information on
supplies and home sprouting)
3 ½ ounces ground chicken breast meat
1 teaspoon dark soy sauce
1 tablespoon light soy sauce, divided
1 tablespoon oyster sauce, divided
1 teaspoon Chinese rice wine (Shao Hsing) or dry sherry
1 tablespoon vegetable oil (soybean, peanut, or canola), divided
2 cloves garlic, chopped, divided
½ cup water or chicken broth, divided
¼ teaspoon salt
¼ teaspoon pepper
1 teaspoon cornstarch
Diced fresh red chili, sliced green onion, and cilantro leaves, as garnish

Wash soybean sprouts; separate white sprouts from the yellow seed
leaves (cotyledons), removing any stringy end roots. Chop seed leaves.
Reserve leaves and sprouts in separate bowls.

Combine chicken, dark soy sauce, 1 teaspoon light soy sauce,
1 teaspoon oyster sauce, and wine in small bowl; let stand 10 minutes.

Heat 2 teaspoons oil in wok over high heat until hot. Sauté half
the garlic until lightly browned, about 1 minute. Stir in white sprouts,
remaining 1 tablespoon light soy sauce, and ¼ cup water; cook
1 minute. Transfer to serving platter, spreading evenly.

Heat remaining 2 teaspoons oil in wok; add remaining garlic. Add
meat mixture and stir-fry 3 minutes; add chopped yellow seed leaves.
Stir well and add remaining 2 teaspoons oyster sauce, salt, and pepper.
Cover and cook 2 minutes.

Combine cornstarch and remaining ¼ cup water in small bowl. Stir into wok, mixing well. Cook 1–2 minutes, until thickened. Spoon pork mixture over cooked sprouts on platter.

Garnish with chili, green onion, and cilantro.

Serves 4.

Note: Serve with salads, noodles, or steamed rice.

Soybean sprouts are rich in vitamin C, phytic acid, and phyto-estrogens. The bright-yellow seed leaves (cotyledons) contain most of the nutrients found in the bean itself, and they are very crunchy in texture and rather nutty in flavor. Trim away the stringy ends and pick off any loose skins of the soybean sprouts before use.

SOYBEAN SPROUTS WITH SHREDDED BEEF

PER SERVING: 161 CALORIES, 15.0 G PROTEIN, 9.7 G CARBOHYDRATE, 8.4 G FAT (1.6 G SATURATED), 408.6 MG SODIUM, 0.8 G FIBER, **PE CONTENT OVER 25 MG**

3 ½ ounces beef tenderloin or strip steak, cut across the grain into thin strips
¾-inch piece gingerroot, finely julienned
1 tablespoon plus 1 teaspoon light soy sauce
2 tablespoons oyster sauce, divided
1 tablespoon plus 1 teaspoon Chinese rice wine (Shao Hsing) or dry sherry
Pinch pepper
½ tablespoon vegetable oil (soybean, peanut, or canola), divided
2 cloves garlic, chopped
4 cups (7 ounces) soybean sprouts, stringy ends trimmed
1 teaspoon cornstarch
⅓ cup water, divided

Combine beef, gingerroot, soy sauce, ½ tablespoon oyster sauce, wine, and pepper in medium bowl; let stand 10 minutes.

Heat 1 teaspoon oil in wok over high heat until hot. Add half the garlic and cook until just starting to brown, about 1 minute. Add soybean sprouts and stir-fry 2 minutes; stir in remaining 1½ tablespoons oyster sauce. Cover wok and continue cooking 2 minutes.

Mix cornstarch and 2 tablespoons water in small bowl. Add to wok and cook, uncovered, 2 minutes. Transfer sprout mixture to serving plate.

Heat remaining oil in wok over high heat until hot. Stir-fry remaining garlic until light brown. Add beef mixture and stir-fry until browned, about 2 minutes. Add remaining 3½ tablespoons water. Cook, covered, 1 minute. Spoon beef over sprouts on serving plate and serve immediately.

Serves 4.

Note: This dish goes well with steamed rice or noodles.

★
★
★
★
★
+

SOYBEAN SPROUTS WITH SHRIMP

PER SERVING: 178 CALORIES, 19.7 G PROTEIN, 8.9 G CARBOHYDRATE, 9.0 G FAT (1.3 G SATURATED), 355.2 MG SODIUM, 0.8 G FIBER, **PE CONTENT OVER 25 MG**

7 ounces shrimp, peeled, deveined
1 tablespoon light soy sauce
1 tablespoon oyster sauce (optional)
1 teaspoon Chinese rice wine or dry sherry
Pinch of pepper
1 tablespoon vegetable oil (soybean, peanut, or canola)
2 cloves garlic, chopped
4 cups (7 ounces) soybean sprouts, stringy ends trimmed
¼ teaspoon salt
1 teaspoon cornstarch
3 tablespoons water
Cilantro leaves, as garnish

Combine shrimp, soy sauce, oyster sauce (if using), wine, and pepper in small bowl; let stand 10 minutes.

Heat oil in wok or large skillet over high heat until hot; add garlic and stir-fry until fragrant, about 1 minute. Add shrimp mixture and stir-fry 2–3 minutes, until pink; remove shrimp from wok and reserve.

Add sprouts to wok; stir-fry about 5 minutes. Return shrimp to wok and stir well. Combine salt, cornstarch, and water in small bowl; stir into wok. Stir until thickened, about 1 minute. Spoon onto serving plate; garnish with cilantro.

Serve hot with boiled rice.

Serves 4.

BAKED SOYBEANS IN EGGPLANT

★
★
★
★
★

PER SERVING: 280 CALORIES, 18.2 G PROTEIN, 24.5 G CARBOHYDRATE, 13.5 G FAT (4.1 G SATURATED), 142.4 MG SODIUM, 8.1 G FIBER, **PE CONTENT 20–25 MG**

1 medium eggplant (10–11 ounces)
1 small onion, chopped
1 clove garlic, chopped
1 teaspoon olive oil
2 ounces lean ground beef or lamb
¼ cup soybeans canned in tomato sauce (if available), or 3 tablespoons soybeans mixed with 1 tablespoon tomato paste and 1 tablespoon water
1 small tomato, diced
⅔ cup small cauliflower florets
Salt and pepper, to taste
3–4 fresh basil leaves, thinly sliced
2 tablespoons grated Parmesan cheese

Preheat oven to 325° F.

Cut eggplant lengthwise and carve out inside of eggplant to form the shape of a boat, leaving ½-inch shell remaining. (Reserve the flesh for another use, such as a vegetable curry.)

Sauté onion and garlic in oil in medium saucepan until light brown, about 3 minutes. Add beef and cook until browned, about 5 minutes. Add soybeans, tomato, and cauliflower, and cook 2 minutes. Season to taste with salt and pepper.

Place eggplant, skin side down, in lightly greased baking dish. Spoon meat mixture into eggplant. Top with basil and cheese. Bake at 325° F for 40 minutes, or until eggplant is soft.

Serve hot with boiled noodles and a green salad.

Serves 2.

Note: Vegetarians may substitute cooked white or brown rice or chopped walnuts for the meat in this recipe.

★
★

STIR-FRIED RICE NOODLES WITH TOFU CUTLET

PER SERVING: 400 CALORIES, 14.0 G PROTEIN, 60.1 G CARBOHYDRATE, 12.1 G FAT (2.0 G SATURATED), 1,171.9 MG SODIUM, 2.4 G FIBER, **PE CONTENT 5–10 MG**

8 ounces rice noodles
2 green onions
1 large egg
½ teaspoon salt
Pinch of pepper
2 tablespoons plus 2 teaspoons vegetable oil (soybean, peanut, canola), divided
2 cloves garlic, chopped
3½ ounces grilled or baked tofu cutlet, cut into strips (see page 92)
3½ ounces peeled, cooked small shrimp, or shredded cooked chicken
2 tablespoons plus 2 teaspoons oyster sauce
4 tablespoons light soy sauce
4 cups (8 ounces) bean sprouts

Soak rice noodles in lukewarm water for 10 minutes, separating strands before draining. Drain well. Chop white parts of green onions; cut stems into 1¼-inch lengths. Set aside in separate bowls.

Beat egg with salt and pepper in small bowl. Heat 1 teaspoon oil in wok over medium heat. When oil is hot, add egg and spread over bottom of wok as if cooking a thin crêpe. When egg is just cooked, remove from the pan—do not overcook egg, as this will make it rubbery. Allow to cool before cutting into ¾-inch strips. Set aside.

Heat remaining 2 tablespoons plus 1 teaspoon oil in wok over high heat until hot. Stir-fry garlic and chopped green onion until light brown. Add cooked shrimp/chicken and tofu and stir-fry 1–2 minutes; add oyster sauce and light soy sauce. Add rice noodles and stir-fry 7–8 minutes. Make a depression in center of noodles and add bean sprouts. Stir-fry 4–5 minutes, adding shrimp during final two minutes. Add cooked egg and green onion stems. Mix well and serve immediately.

Serves 4.

STIR-FRIED CHINESE CABBAGE AND BEAN THREAD NOODLES

★

PER SERVING: 120 CALORIES, 4.01 G PROTEIN, 12.4 G CARBOHYDRATE, 6.0 G FAT (0.7 G SATURATED), 420.4 MG SODIUM, 1.6 G FIBER, **PE CONTENT 0–5 MG**

2 ounces bean thread noodles (cellophane vermicelli)
3½ ounces ground chicken breast meat
2 teaspoons Chinese rice wine (Shao Hsing) or dry sherry
2 tablespoons plus 2 teaspoons oyster sauce, divided
1 tablespoon plus 1 teaspoon light soy sauce
¼ teaspoon pepper
2 tablespoons vegetable oil (soybean, peanut, canola)
2 cloves garlic, chopped
½ small head (8 ounces) of Chinese (Napa) cabbage, sliced
1 medium carrot, shredded
¼ teaspoon salt
1 teaspoon cornstarch
½ cup water

Soak noodles in cold water for 20 minutes. Drain well and cut into lengths 4–6 inches long. Set aside.

Combine chicken meat, wine, 1 tablespoon oyster sauce, soy sauce, and pepper in small bowl; let stand 15–20 minutes.

Heat oil in wok over high heat until hot; stir-fry garlic until fragrant, about 1 minute. Immediately stir in chicken. Stir-fry 3–4 minutes, or until light brown. Add Chinese cabbage and stir-fry 2–3 minutes. Add carrot and noodles. Stir well and cook 3–4 minutes. Add remaining 1 tablespoon plus 2 teaspoons oyster sauce and salt.

Combine cornstarch and water in small bowl; stir into wok. Cook until thickened, about 2 minutes.

Serve with other stir-fried vegetables and steamed rice.

Serves 6.

Bean thread noodles, available from the Asian section of many supermarkets, are made from mung bean flour and are rich in proteins and B vitamins. They also contain phytoestrogens. Besides stir-fries, bean threads can also be used in soups. When deep fried (without soaking) they puff up and expand spectacularly, making a wonderful crisp topping for stir-fries.

MEDITERRANEAN SPINACH PASTA

★
★
★
★
★
★
+

PER SERVING: 396 CALORIES, 20.4 G PROTEIN, 14.1 G CARBOHYDRATE, 12.2 G FAT (1.4 G
SATURATED), 284.6 MG SODIUM, 4.8 G FIBER, **PE CONTENT OVER 25 MG**

1 tablespoon olive oil
14 ounces firm tofu, cut into ¾-inch cubes
1 small onion, chopped
1 red bell pepper, cut into 1-inch pieces
2 medium zucchini, sliced ¼-inch thick
1 can (14½ ounces) no-salt-added cut tomatoes, undrained
8 pitted black olives or green Spanish olives, sliced
1 package (about 9 ounces) fresh spinach pasta, cooked, warm

Heat oil in large nonstick skillet over medium-high heat until hot.
Sauté tofu until lightly browned; remove from pan and set aside. Add
onion, bell pepper, and zucchini to pan; sauté 3 minutes. Return tofu
to pan; add tomatoes and liquid, and olives. Cover and simmer until
vegetables are barely tender, 5–7 minutes. Toss with pasta.

Serves 4.

Recipe from *Delicious and Easy Recipes for Tofu and Pasta.* By permission of Azumaya.

★
★
★
★

SESAME TOFU AND SPINACH PASTA

PER SERVING: 452 CALORIES, 21.7 G PROTEIN, 61.0 G CARBOHYDRATE, 14.2 G FAT (2.4 G SATURATED), 435.0 MG SODIUM, 5.3 G FIBER, **PE CONTENT 15–20 MG**

7 ounces extra-firm tofu (or baked tofu cutlet; see page 92)
2 tablespoons light soy sauce
4 teaspoons sesame seeds
4 teaspoons olive oil, divided
2 cloves garlic, minced
12 asparagus spears, cut into 1-inch lengths
1 yellow bell pepper, cut into strips
7 cherry tomatoes, cut into halves
1 tablespoon Asian chili sauce or chili oil, or to taste
1 package (about 9 ounces) fresh spinach pasta, cooked, warm

Place tofu on plate, and lay another plate on top of it. Place a 28-ounce (or similar weight) can on top plate. Let tofu stand under weight for about an hour or overnight in refrigerator. This will make it very firm. (This step may be omitted if using baked tofu cutlet.)

Dry tofu, cut into strips, and toss with soy sauce and sesame seeds in small bowl.

Heat 2 teaspoons olive oil in medium nonstick skillet over medium heat until hot. Add tofu mixture and sauté, turning gently, until golden brown on all sides. Set aside.

Sauté remaining 2 teaspoons olive oil and garlic in large nonstick skillet until fragrant, about 1 minute. Add asparagus and yellow bell pepper and sauté about 5 minutes, or until just tender. Add cherry tomatoes and sauté 2 minutes.

Combine tofu, vegetables, chili sauce, and pasta in medium bowl; toss well and serve immediately.

Serves 3.

Recipe from *Delicious and Easy Recipes for Tofu and Pasta*. By permission of Azumaya.

EASY VEGETABLE LASAGNA

★
★

PER SERVING: 286 CALORIES, 16.4 G PROTEIN, 38.8 G CARBOHYDRATE, 7.8 G FAT (3.3 G SATURATED),
1,154.4 MG SODIUM, 6.1 G FIBER, **PE CONTENT 5–10 MG**

8 green onions, chopped
1 cup sliced mushrooms
1 tablespoon olive oil
1 clove garlic, minced
1 jar (48 ounces) spaghetti sauce
½ package (10½-ounce size)
low-fat firm silken tofu
1 package (10 ounces) frozen
chopped spinach, thawed, drained
1 egg
½ teaspoon salt

¼ teaspoon pepper
½ teaspoon dried oregano leaves
1 tablespoon chopped fresh,
or ½ teaspoon dried, basil leaves
1 package (8 ounces) no-boil
lasagna noodles, or regular lasagna
noodles, cooked
1 ball (8 ounces) part-skim
mozzarella, shredded
¼ cup grated Parmesan cheese
(optional)

Preheat oven to 350° F.

Sauté green onions and mushrooms in olive oil over medium heat until mushrooms are browned. Add garlic and stir briefly until translucent. Add spaghetti sauce and set aside.

Combine tofu, spinach, egg, and seasonings in medium bowl and mix well.

Spoon half the spaghetti-sauce mixture in bottom of lightly greased 9 x 13–inch baking dish. Top with half the noodles, half of the mozzarella cheese, tofu mixture, and remaining noodles; top with remaining sauce. Cover lasagna tightly with aluminum foil and bake at 350° F for 45 minutes. Remove foil and sprinkle remaining cheeses on top. Bake, uncovered, 15 minutes or until cheese is melted and browned. Let stand at room temperature 10 minutes before serving.

Serves 8–10.

Recipe adapted from a recipe reprinted courtesy of the Indiana Soybean Board.

★
★
★
★
★
+

Tuna Soy-Mac Casserole

PER SERVING WITH SOY CHEESE: 493 CALORIES, 36.3 G PROTEIN, 47.2 G CARBOHYDRATE, 16.4 G FAT
(2.4 G SATURATED), 1,110.6 MG SODIUM, 3.5 G FIBER.

PER SERVING WITH CHEDDAR CHEESE: 569 CALORIES, 38.1 G PROTEIN, 46.1 G CARBOHYDRATE,
25.8 G FAT (12.0 G SATURATED), 1,085.1 MG SODIUM, 3.5 G FIBER, **PE CONTENT 20–25 MG**

2 medium onions, divided
1 tablespoon olive oil
1 can (7 ounces) water-packed tuna,
    drained
10 ounces low-fat silken tofu
1½ cups water, divided
½ teaspoon salt

½ teaspoon pepper
1 teaspoon onion powder
1 tablespoon plus 1 teaspoon
    cornstarch
7 ounces soy macaroni, cooked
2 medium tomatoes, sliced
1¾ cups (7 ounces) shredded
    Cheddar cheese, or soy cheese

Preheat oven to 350° F.

Chop 1 onion and sauté in oil in large saucepan until tender, about 5 minutes. Stir in tuna.

Blend tofu with ¾ cup water. Add tofu mixture, salt, pepper, and onion powder to saucepan. Add ½ cup water; heat to boiling. Mix cornstarch with remaining ¼ cup water and stir into saucepan, stirring constantly until thickened. Stir in macaroni.

Slice remaining onion and arrange in lightly greased 2-quart casserole. Pour half the pasta mixture over onion. Arrange tomatoes on top of pasta, and cover with remaining pasta mixture. Sprinkle with cheese.

Bake, covered, at 350° F until hot and bubbly, about 20 minutes.

Serve hot, accompanied by a garden salad.

Serves 4.

Note: Soy milk can be used instead of tofu in this dish. Reduce the amount of water to ¼ cup. Add 1¾ cups soy milk to tuna, along with salt, pepper, and onion powder. Thicken with cornstarch and water mixture, and complete recipe as written.

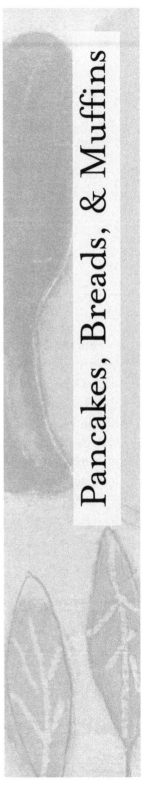

Pancakes, Breads, & Muffins

★
★
★
★

Soy Pancakes

PER SERVING: 175 CALORIES, 6.3 G PROTEIN, 26.6 G CARBOHYDRATE, 5.1 G FAT (0.8 G SATURATED), 322.3 MG SODIUM, 1.6 G FIBER, **PE CONTENT 15–20 MG**

½ cup soy flour
1 cup all-purpose flour
½ teaspoon salt
1¼ teaspoons baking powder
1 large egg, beaten
2 tablespoons plus 2 teaspoons sugar
1 cup low-fat soy milk
1 tablespoon cooking oil, divided

Sift soy flour, all-purpose flour, salt, and baking powder together into large bowl. Make a well in center and stir in combined egg, sugar, soy milk, and ½ tablespoon oil. Mix until smooth.

Heat remaining ½ tablespoon oil in large skillet or griddle over medium-high heat until hot. Spoon about 2 tablespoons batter for each pancake into pan. When pancakes are golden brown on bottoms, turn and cook until golden brown on the other side. Repeat with remaining batter.

Serve with your favorite jam and freshly whipped cream. Or top with fat-free yogurt and fresh fruit if you're watching your fat intake.

Serves 6.

BANANA OAT PANCAKES

★
★
★
★

PER SERVING: 150 CALORIES, 4.8 G PROTEIN, 26.2 G CARBOHYDRATE, 3.6G FAT (0.8 G SATURATED), 233.6 MG SODIUM, 2.2 G FIBER, **PE CONTENT 10–15 MG**

½ cup rolled oats
½ cup unbleached flour
¼ cup soy flour
1 tablespoon baking powder
1½ cups plain soy milk
2 bananas, thinly sliced

Combine rolled oats, unbleached flour, soy flour, and baking powder in large bowl. Mix in soy milk, stirring until smooth. Fold in banana slices.

Heat nonstick griddle or pan over medium-high heat until hot. Pour in ¼ cup batter. Cook about 2 minutes or until bubbles appear on surface. Turn pancake and cook until browned on other side and heated through, about 1 minute. Repeat with remaining batter.

Serve pancakes with maple syrup, fruit spread, or applesauce.

Makes 6 servings of 2 pancakes each.

Recipe courtesy of the Indiana Soybean Board.

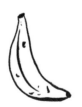

★

CRUSTY SOY BREAD

PER SLICE: 111 CALORIES, 4.0 G PROTEIN, 20.6 G CARBOHYDRATE, 1.3 G FAT (0.2 G SATURATED), 107.5 MG SODIUM, 1.1 G FIBER, **PE CONTENT 0–5 MG**

2½ cups bread flour
½ cup soy flour
1 teaspoon salt
1 teaspoon sugar
1 package dry yeast
½ cup plain soy milk, warm
½ cup warm water (105°–115° F)

Conventional Method:

Preheat oven to 350° F.

Mix dry ingredients together in large mixing bowl. Gradually add liquids and knead dough 2–3 minutes. Place dough in lightly greased bowl and turn to coat dough. Cover with waxed paper and a towel. Let rise in a warm place until doubled in size, about one hour. On lightly floured surface, punch down several times to remove air bubbles. Shape into loaf. Place in 5 x 7–inch loaf pan. Cover, place in a warm spot, and let rise 45 minutes or until almost doubled in size. Bake at 350° F for 30–40 minutes, or until bread is golden and sounds hollow when tapped. Remove from pan and cool on wire rack or serve immediately.

Bread Machine Method:

Add ingredients to bread machine according to manufacturer's instructions. All ingredients should be at room temperature. Use the crusty-bread setting for French bread.

Makes one 1½-pound loaf (approximately 14 slices).

Note: This bread will not rise as high as traditional breads.

Recipe from *It's Soy Easy…to Cook with Soy.* By permission of the Ohio Soybean Council.

HERB AND CHEESE FOCACCIA ★ ★

PER SERVING: 223 CALORIES, 10.7 G PROTEIN, 34.6 G CARBOHYDRATE, 4.6 G FAT (1.7 G SATURATED), 449.7 MG SODIUM, 2.3 G FIBER, **PE CONTENT 5–10 MG**

1 package rapid-rise dry yeast
1 teaspoon sugar
¾ cup warm water (105°–115° F)
½ cup (2 ounces) shredded Parmesan cheese, divided
1 teaspoon seasoned salt
1 teaspoon garlic powder
1¼ teaspoons dried Italian seasoning blend
2 cups all-purpose flour
¼ cup soy flour
Vegetable oil, for brushing

Preheat oven to 375° F.

Sprinkle yeast and sugar over warm water in small bowl; stir to dissolve and set aside. Place ¼ cup Parmesan cheese, salt, garlic powder, Italian seasoning, and flours in food processor and process 4–5 seconds, until well blended. With processor running, slowly add yeast mixture through feed tube; process until dough forms a ball, about 45 seconds. Dough will be slightly sticky. Place dough in lightly greased bowl and turn once to coat. Cover. Let rise in a warm place until doubled in size, about 45 minutes. Punch down.

Roll dough on lightly floured surface into 12-inch circle and place on pizza stone or pan. Brush with oil. Let rise 15 minutes.

Bake at 375° F for 18–20 minutes, or until light brown. Sprinkle with remaining ¼ cup cheese. Return to oven for 3 minutes, or until cheese melts.

Serves 6.

Focaccia Pizza: Before baking, add toppings such as sliced vegetables, mushrooms, grilled chicken, low-fat sausage, or soy meat, and top with sliced skim-milk mozzarella and additional Parmesan cheese.

Recipe from *It's Soy Easy…to Cook with Soy*. By permission of the Ohio Soybean Council.

CHERRY MUFFINS

PER MUFFIN: 189 CALORIES, 4.8 G PROTEIN, 31.8 G CARBOHYDRATE, 5.6 G FAT (0.8 G SATURATED), 194.0 MG SODIUM, 2.1 G FIBER, **PE CONTENT 5–10 MG**

¾ cup packed light brown sugar
1 tablespoon plus 1 teaspoon honey
¼ cup plus 1 tablespoon canola oil
2 large eggs, beaten
½ cup soy flour
1 cup whole-wheat flour
1½ teaspoons baking powder
½ teaspoon salt
⅔ cup plain soy milk
1 cup pitted cherries, halved

Preheat oven to 350° F.

Mix brown sugar, honey, and oil in large mixing bowl. Add eggs and mix well. Stir in combined soy flour, whole-wheat flour, baking powder, and salt. Add soy milk and stir until batter is smooth. Fold in cherries.

Spoon batter into lightly greased muffin tins. Bake at 350° F until muffins are browned and toothpick inserted in center of muffins comes out clean, about 20 minutes.

Cool muffins in pan 5 minutes; remove and cool on wire rack.

Makes 10–12 regular or 28–30 mini muffins.

Muffins will keep for a few days if stored in an airtight container.

Canned pitted cherries can be used in this recipe. Cherries contain phytoestrogens. The batter may smell a little odd when wet because of the soy flour, but the smell invariably disappears with cooking.

APPLE MUFFINS

★
★

PER MUFFIN: 208 CALORIES, 4.8 G PROTEIN, 33.6 G CARBOHYDRATE, 7.1 G FAT (0.9 G SATURATED),
195.8 MG SODIUM, 2.3 G FIBER, **PE CONTENT 5–10 MG**

2 apples (7 ounces), peeled and diced
¾ cup packed light brown sugar
1 tablespoon plus 1 teaspoon honey
⅓ cup canola oil
2 eggs, beaten
½ cup soy flour
1 cup whole-wheat flour
1½ teaspoons baking powder
2 teaspoons ground cinnamon
½ teaspoon salt
⅔ cup soy milk

Preheat oven to 350° F.

Microwave apple in small dish at high until soft, about 4 minutes. Cool.

Mix brown sugar, honey, oil, and eggs in large bowl. Sift soy flour, whole-wheat flour, baking powder, cinnamon, and salt into bowl and stir well. Gradually mix in soy milk. When batter is smooth, fold in apple.

Spoon batter into lightly greased muffin tins. Bake at 350° F until muffins are browned and toothpick inserted in center of muffins comes out clean, about 20 minutes. (Regular muffins require about 21 minutes, while small muffins require about 18 minutes baking time.)

Cool muffins in pan 5 minutes; remove and cool on wire rack.

Makes 10–12 regular or 28–30 mini muffins.

> Eggs can be omitted from this recipe and extra soy milk
> used in their place. Substitute 1 tablespoon plus 1 teaspoon
> soy milk for each egg. The honey and soy flour give these
> muffins a very moist texture.

★
★

BANANA OATMEAL MUFFINS

PER MUFFIN: 159 CALORIES, 4.4 G PROTEIN, 27.5 G CARBOHYDRATE, 4.0 G FAT (0.6 G SATURATED),
250.5 MG SODIUM, 1.9 G FIBER, **PE CONTENT 5–10 MG**

1 cup old-fashioned rolled oats
¾ cup unbleached flour
½ cup soy flour
½ cup sugar
1 tablespoon baking powder
½ teaspoon baking soda
½ teaspoon salt
3 medium very ripe bananas
1 cup plain yogurt or soy yogurt
2 tablespoons vegetable oil
½ cup flaked or shredded coconut (optional)

Preheat oven to 375° F.

Process oats in food processor or blender until oats are the texture of coarse flour. Add flours, sugar, baking powder, baking soda, and salt, and process briefly to combine. Transfer to large mixing bowl.

Process bananas in food processor until coarsely mashed. Add yogurt and oil and process until smooth. Stir banana mixture into flour mixture, stirring just until mixed. (Batter will be thick.)

Spoon batter into lightly greased muffin tins. Sprinkle with coconut, if desired. Bake at 375° F until muffins are browned and toothpick inserted in center of muffins comes out clean, about 20 minutes.

Cool muffins in pan 5 minutes; remove and cool on wire rack. Makes 12 muffins.

Recipe from Laura Nilsen, highlighted in *Veggie Life* (January 1999).

SWEET POTATO MUFFINS ★

PER MUFFIN: 167 CALORIES, 3.7 G PROTEIN, 32.4 G CARBOHYDRATE, 3.0 G FAT (0.4 G SATURATED),
278.8 MG SODIUM, 2.4 G FIBER, **PE CONTENT 0–5 MG**

1 cup unbleached flour
1 cup whole-wheat flour
1 tablespoon baking powder
½ teaspoon baking soda
1 teaspoon grated orange rind
½ teaspoon salt
¼ teaspoon ground nutmeg
1 cup cooked sweet potatoes
½ cup sugar
¼ cup orange juice
2 tablespoons vegetable oil
1 tablespoon molasses
1 cup plain soy milk
¼ cup finely chopped pecans (optional)
2 tablespoons brown sugar (optional)

Preheat oven to 375° F.

Combine flours, baking powder, baking soda, orange rind, salt, and nutmeg in large bowl. Process sweet potato in food processor until mashed. Add sugar, orange juice, oil, and molasses; process until mixed. Gradually add soy milk and process until smooth. Stir sweet potato mixture into flour mixture, stirring just until mixed.

Spoon batter into lightly greased muffin tins. If desired, combine pecans and brown sugar in small bowl; sprinkle over muffins. Bake at 375° F until muffins are browned and toothpick inserted in center of muffins comes out clean, about 20 minutes.

Cool muffins in pan 5 minutes; remove and cool on wire rack.

Makes 12 muffins.

Recipe from Laura Nilsen, highlighted in *Veggie Life* (January 1999).

★ LITTLE LEMON AND GREEN TEA MUFFINS

PER MUFFIN: 56 CALORIES, 1.6 G PROTEIN, 8.8 G CARBOHYDRATE, 1.6 G FAT (0.2 G SATURATED),
107.1 MG SODIUM, 0.3 G FIBER, **PE CONTENT 0–5 MG**

1⅓ cups unbleached flour
⅓ cup soy flour
⅓ cup sugar
1 tablespoon loose green tea, ground in coffee grinder or spice grinder
2 teaspoons baking powder
½ teaspoon baking soda
½ teaspoon salt
1 cup lemon-flavored yogurt or soy yogurt
2 tablespoons vegetable oil
⅓ cup water or soy milk
½ teaspoon grated lemon rind
2 tablespoons mild honey (optional)
2 teaspoons lemon juice (optional)

Preheat oven to 375° F.

Combine flours, sugar, ground tea, baking powder, baking soda, and salt in large bowl. Combine yogurt, oil, water, and lemon rind in small bowl. Stir yogurt mixture into flour mixture, stirring just until smooth.

Spoon batter into lightly greased mini-muffin tins. Bake at 375° F until muffins are browned and toothpick inserted in center of muffins comes out clean, about 20 minutes.

If desired, combine honey and lemon juice in small bowl. Drizzle glaze over hot muffins before removing from muffin pans.

Cool muffins in pan 5 minutes; remove and cool on wire rack.

Makes 24 mini-muffins.

Recipe from Laura Nilsen, highlighted in *Veggie Life* (January 1999).

DOUBLE CHOCOLATE MUFFINS

★
★
★

PER MUFFIN: 190 CALORIES, 4.1 G PROTEIN, 32.6 G CARBOHYDRATE, 4.2 G FAT (0.8 G SATURATED), 393.0 MG SODIUM, 1.6 G FIBER, **PE CONTENT 10–15 MG**

1½ cups unbleached flour
½ cup soy flour
1 cup packed light brown sugar
⅓ cup unsweetened cocoa
1 tablespoon baking powder
1 teaspoon baking soda
1 teaspoon salt
1 cup chocolate-flavored soy milk
½ cup plain yogurt or soy yogurt
2 tablespoons vegetable oil
1 teaspoon vanilla
½ cup sliced almonds (optional)

Preheat oven to 375° F.

Combine flours, brown sugar, cocoa, baking powder, baking soda, and salt in large bowl. Whisk soy milk, yogurt, oil, and vanilla in small bowl until smooth. Stir soy-milk mixture into flour mixture, stirring just until mixed.

Spoon batter into lightly greased muffin tins. Sprinkle with almonds, if desired. Bake at 375° F until muffins are browned and toothpick inserted in center of muffins comes out clean, about 20 minutes.

Cool muffins in pan 5 minutes; remove and cool on wire rack.

Makes 12 muffins.

Recipe from Laura Nilsen, highlighted in *Veggie Life* (January 1999).

★
★
★

Fruity Soy Scones

PER SERVING: 255 CALORIES, 7.1 G PROTEIN, 38.7 G CARBOHYDRATE, 8.2 G FAT (4.0 G SATURATED),
704.6 MG SODIUM, 2.7 G FIBER, **PE CONTENT 10–15 MG**

1 ¼ cups self-rising flour
¼ cup soy flour
½ teaspoon baking powder
¼ teaspoon baking soda
2 tablespoons butter, softened
¼ cup soy milk
3 ounces apricot or other fruit-flavored soy yogurt
2 tablespoons diced dried apricots
1 tablespoon dried dark raisins

Preheat oven to 375° F.

Sift the flours, baking powder, and baking soda into medium bowl; cut in butter until mixture resembles coarse crumbs.

Mix soy milk and yogurt in small bowl; add to flour mixture.

Knead lightly with oiled hands, and add fruits. Place dough on floured pastry board; shape dough into a round about 1 to 1¼ inches thick. Cut into smaller rounds with 2-inch cookie or biscuit cutter. Place on lightly greased baking sheet and bake at 375° F until golden brown, about 18 minutes.

Serve warm, cut into halves, with fruit jams.

Makes 4 servings of 2 scones each.

SOY AND DATE SCONES

★
★
★
★

PER SERVING: 309 CALORIES, 10.3 G PROTEIN, 44.5 G CARBOHYDRATE, 12.0 G FAT
(5.8 G SATURATED), 265.4 MG SODIUM, 6.8 G FIBER, **PE CONTENT 15–20 MG**

¼ cup butter or margarine, softened
2 cups whole-wheat flour
½ cup soy flour
2 teaspoons baking powder
2 tablespoons packed light brown sugar
1 egg, lightly beaten
⅓ cup chopped pitted dates
1 cup soy milk

Preheat oven to 400° F.

Beat butter on low speed of cake mixer until light. In a separate bowl, combine whole-wheat flour, soy flour, and baking powder; add to butter. Add sugar, egg, dates, and soy milk.

Place dough on floured pastry board and knead lightly; shape dough into a round about 1 to 1¼ inches thick. Cut into smaller rounds with 2-inch cookie or biscuit cutter. Place on lightly greased baking sheet and bake at 400° F until golden brown, about 12 minutes.

Serve with fruit jam.

Makes 6 servings of 2 scones each.

Recipe from Mrs. G. Hathaway.

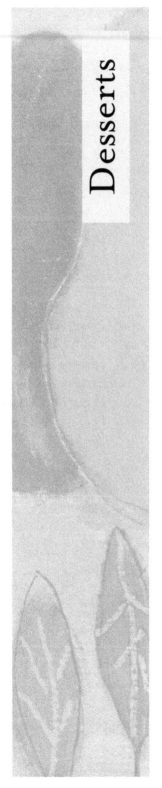

Desserts

STRAWBERRY SOY DESSERT

PER SERVING: 147 CALORIES, 4.6 G PROTEIN, 20.8 G CARBOHYDRATE, 4.4 G FAT (1.0 G SATURATED), 100.8 MG SODIUM, 1.9 G FIBER, **PE CONTENT 10–15 MG**

1 cup soy milk
1 cup strawberry halves
4 teaspoons sugar
2 teaspoons strawberry-flavored milk drink mix
(such as Nestle's Strawberry Quik)
1 envelope unflavored gelatin
¼ cup water

Process soy milk and strawberries in blender until smooth; add sugar and drink mix and blend 30 seconds.

Sprinkle gelatin over water in medium saucepan; let stand until softened, about 2 minutes. Stir over medium heat until gelatin has dissolved completely. Add strawberry mixture to saucepan, stirring well.

Pour into 2 dessert bowls and refrigerate several hours, until set. Serves 2.

Gelatin has a high protein content.

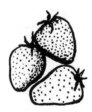

Banana Berry Whip

★
★
★
★
★
★

PER SERVING: 175 CALORIES, 4.8 G PROTEIN, 16.4 G CARBOHYDRATE, 2.4 G FAT (0.1 G SATURATED), 0.7 MG SODIUM, 3.1 G FIBER, **PE CONTENT 20–25 MG**

¼ cup fresh or frozen raspberries
¼ cup fresh or frozen strawberries
1 medium banana
4–6 ice cubes (omit if using frozen berries)
2 cups vanilla-flavored soy milk

Process all ingredients in blender until thick and smooth.
Serves 2–3.

Recipe from *Healthy and Delicious Recipes, Vol. 1.* By permission of VitaSoy.

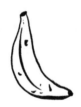

★
★
★

BAKED HONEY CUSTARD

PER SERVING: 363 CALORIES, 10.7 G PROTEIN, 51.2 G CARBOHYDRATE, 13.6 G FAT
(3.5 G SATURATED), 380.8 MG SODIUM, 0.1 G FIBER, **PE CONTENT 10–15 MG**

2 cups plain soy milk
2 eggs, lightly beaten
¼ cup honey
1 teaspoon vanilla
⅛ teaspoon salt
Cinnamon sugar

Preheat oven to 300° F.

Whisk soy milk, eggs, honey, vanilla, and salt in medium bowl. Pour mixture into 4 custard cups or a 1-quart soufflé dish. Place cups or soufflé dish in larger pan; place pan on oven rack and pour in boiling water halfway up sides of cups or dish.

Bake at 300° F until knife inserted near edge of custard comes out clean, about 20 minutes. Cool; refrigerate until cold, about 1 hour. Custard will firm as it cools. Sprinkle with cinnamon sugar.

Serves 4–6.

Recipe from *Healthy and Delicious Recipes, Vol. 1.* By permission of VitaSoy.

SOY AND OATMEAL COOKIES ★

PER COOKIE: 93 CALORIES, 2.1 G PROTEIN, 12.5 G CARBOHYDRATE, 3.8 G FAT (2.0 G SATURATED), 54.2 MG SODIUM, 1.2 G FIBER, **PE CONTENT 0–5 MG**

½ cup butter, softened
¾ cup packed light brown sugar
1 large egg
2 teaspoons vanilla
½ cup low-fat plain soy milk
½ cup soy flour
½ cup all-purpose flour
½ teaspoon baking soda
2 teaspoons ground cinnamon
2½ cups quick-cooking oats

Preheat oven to 325° F.

Cream butter and brown sugar in medium mixer bowl until fluffy; beat in egg and vanilla, beating until smooth. Beat in soy milk.

Sift flours, baking soda, and cinnamon together. Add to creamed mixture and mix well; stir in oats.

Roll about 1 tablespoon dough into ball with lightly greased hands; press dough flat and place on lightly greased baking sheet. Repeat with remaining dough. Bake at 325° F until lightly browned, about 20 minutes. Remove cookies from baking sheets immediately and cool on wire rack.

Makes about 28 cookies.

Five of these cookies contain approximately the same amount of phytoestrogens as 3½ fluid ounces of high-protein soy milk.

Soy flour keeps better if stored in an airtight container in the refrigerator. Soy flour is heavier than wheat flour and retains a lot of moisture after baking. Rolled oats are very rich in fiber and also contain phytoestrogens.

★ ★ ★ BANANA-TOPPED CHOCOLATE SILK PIE

PER SERVING: 306 CALORIES, 5.4 G PROTEIN, 34.5 G CARBOHYDRATE, 18.2 G FAT (7.8 G SATURATED), 99.4 MG SODIUM, 3.3 G FIBER, **PE CONTENT 10–15 MG**

12 ounces semisweet or dark chocolate, chopped
12 ounces soft silken tofu
1 teaspoon vanilla
1 pie shell (9 inch), baked
2 medium bananas, thinly sliced
¼ cup (2 ounces) melted semisweet chocolate, as garnish
¼ cup chopped pistachios, as garnish

Melt chopped chocolate in top of double boiler over hot water, stirring frequently. While chocolate is melting, process tofu in food processor or blender until smooth; add chocolate and process until completely blended. Add vanilla and pulse to blend.

Pour chocolate mixture into baked pie shell, spreading with spatula. Refrigerate, covered, until set, about 60 minutes. Arrange bananas on top of pie; drizzle with melted chocolate and sprinkle with pistachios. Let pie stand at room temperature 15 minutes before serving.

Serves 10.

Recipe created by Dana Jacob; adapted from *Delicious and Easy Recipes for Tofu and Pasta*. By permission of Azumaya.

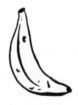

HEART-HEALTHY PUMPKIN PIE ★ ★ ★

PER SERVING: 269 CALORIES, 5.6 G PROTEIN, 41.6 G CARBOHYDRATE, 10.2 G FAT (2.4 G SATURATED),
241.5 MG SODIUM, 2.7 G FIBER, **PE CONTENT 5–10 MG**

1 unbaked 9-inch pie shell
10 ounces firm tofu
½ cup granulated sugar
¼ cup packed light brown sugar
1 teaspoon ground cinnamon
½ teaspoon ground ginger
½ teaspoon ground nutmeg
¼ teaspoon ground cloves
½ teaspoon salt
1 teaspoon vanilla
1 large egg (optional)
1 can (16 ounces) pumpkin

Preheat oven to 400° F.

Pierce bottom and sides of pie shell with fork. Bake at 400° F for
10 minutes. If shell puffs during baking, pierce with fork, and return to
oven. (Shell may also be baked filled with pie weights, dried beans, or
rice to keep it from puffing.)

Process tofu, granulated sugar, brown sugar, spices, salt, vanilla, and
egg (if using) in food processor or blender until smooth. Strain through
wire strainer placed over large bowl. Whisk in pumpkin. Spoon filling
into pie shell, spreading evenly. Bake at 400° F for 15 minutes. Reduce
oven heat to 350° F and bake 40 minutes longer, or until set.

Cool on wire rack; serve warm, or refrigerate and serve chilled.

Serves 8.

Recipe from *Delicious and Easy Recipes for Tofu and Pasta*. By permission of Azumaya.

SOY APPLE CAKE

PER SERVING: 274 CALORIES, 5.0 G PROTEIN, 32.6 G CARBOHYDRATE, 14.8 G FAT (2.2 G SATURATED), 277.9 MG SODIUM, 3.5 G FIBER, **PE CONTENT 10–15 MG**

4 medium green apples, peeled, thinly sliced
1 teaspoon ground cinnamon
4 whole cloves
½ cup sugar, divided
½ cup all-purpose flour
½ cup defatted soy flour

1¼ teaspoons baking powder
¼ teaspoon baking soda
½ teaspoon salt
½ cup soybean or canola oil
1 egg
⅔ cup lite soy milk
¼ cup shredded coconut (optional)

Preheat oven to 325° F.

Combine apples, cinnamon, cloves, and 1 tablespoon sugar in microwave-safe dish. Microwave for 4 minutes, or until apples are softened; cool. Discard cloves.

Sift flour, soy flour, baking powder, baking soda, and salt together into small bowl. Beat remaining 7 tablespoons sugar, oil, and egg in medium bowl. Fold in flour mixture; add soy milk and stir until smooth.

Place cooled apples in lightly greased deep 9-inch round cake pan. Spoon cake batter over apples.

Sprinkle ¼ cup shredded coconut (if using) evenly over the top (see note below).

Bake at 325° F for 50–60 minutes, or until a skewer inserted into the center of cake comes out clean. Cut the cake into 8 wedges and serve warm.

Serves 8.

Note: Nutritional information does not include shredded coconut. Although it improves the flavor of this cake greatly, it will increase the fat content of this recipe. Canned cherries or seeded prunes can be used instead of fresh apples.

SOY CARROT CAKE

★
★
★

PER SERVING: 340 CALORIES, 4.7 G PROTEIN, 30.9 G CARBOHYDRATE, 23.0 G FAT (3.1 G SATURATED), 337.3 MG SODIUM, 1.8 G FIBER, **PE CONTENT 5–10 MG**

½ cup soy flour
½ cup wheat flour
1½ teaspoons baking powder
½ teaspoon baking soda
1½ teaspoons ground cinnamon
½ teaspoon salt

⅔ cup vegetable oil
¾ cup sugar
2 eggs
½ cup crushed pineapple
1 cup shredded carrots
¼ cup chopped pecans

Preheat oven to 350° F.

Sift soy flour, wheat flour, baking powder, baking soda, cinnamon, and salt together into small bowl.

Beat oil, sugar, and eggs in medium bowl until light and fluffy. Gradually add flour mixture, stirring until well mixed. Stir in remaining ingredients. Pour into greased 9-inch round or 8-inch square cake pan.

Bake at 350° F for 50–60 minutes, or until a skewer inserted into the center of the cake comes out clean. Cool in pan on wire rack 10 minutes; invert onto wire rack to cool completely.

Serves 8.

Note: If you want to frost this cake, to make Cream Cheese Frosting, beat together ¼ cup butter, ½ teaspoon vanilla extract, and 4 ounces (½ cup) cream cheese. Slowly add 1½ cups confectioners' (icing) sugar to the creamed mixture, beating continuously, until you reach the desired consistency.

Recipe adapted from an original recipe by Mrs. Sherry Jordan.

Frosting is very sweet and high in calories, so simply leave the cake unfrosted if you are on a weight-reduction program.

★
★

Soy Tea Cake

PER SERVING: 235 CALORIES, 5.3 G PROTEIN, 36.6 G CARBOHYDRATE, 7.8 G FAT (3.8 G SATURATED),
421.7 MG SODIUM, 1.5 G FIBER, **PE CONTENT 5–10 MG**

2 tablespoons butter or margarine, softened
½ cup packed light brown sugar
Pinch of salt
1 egg, well beaten
½ cup soy milk
¼ teaspoon vanilla
1 cup self-rising whole-meal flour
⅓ cup soy flour
1 teaspoon baking powder
2 teaspoons melted butter or margarine
1 teaspoon ground cinnamon
1 teaspoon granulated sugar

Preheat oven to 325° F.

Beat butter, brown sugar, and salt in mixing bowl until smooth. Add egg, soy milk, and vanilla. Combine whole-meal flour, soy flour, and baking powder; stir into butter mixture. Pour into lightly greased 5 x 7–inch loaf pan.

Bake at 325° F for 30–35 minutes, or until skewer comes out clean. Remove from baking pan and brush with melted butter while still hot. Sprinkle with combined cinnamon and granulated sugar.

Serves 6.

Adapted from a recipe provided by Mrs. G. Hathaway.

Soy Bread and Butter Pudding

★
★
★
★
★
★

PER SERVING: 351 CALORIES, 8.3 G PROTEIN, 49.5 G CARBOHYDRATE, 13.9 G FAT (6.7 G SATURATED), 367.2 MG SODIUM, 2.5 G FIBER, **PE CONTENT 20–25 MG**

6 slices soy and linseed bread, crusts removed
3 tablespoons butter, softened
⅓ cup dark raisins
1½ cups lite soy milk
2 eggs
1 teaspoon vanilla
¼ cup packed brown sugar, divided
1 teaspoon ground cinnamon, divided
½ teaspoon ground nutmeg

Preheat oven to 350° F.

Spread bread lightly on both sides with butter. Arrange bread in layers in lightly greased 8 x 8–inch baking dish, sprinkling raisins between layers.

Whisk soy milk, eggs, vanilla, 3 tablespoons brown sugar, and ½ teaspoon cinnamon in medium bowl. Pour over bread and press down to moisten bread.

Combine remaining 1 tablespoon brown sugar, ½ teaspoon cinnamon, and nutmeg in small bowl. Sprinkle over top of bread pudding.

Place baking dish in larger deep baking pan. Fill pan with 1 inch hot water. Bake at 350° F until set, about 50 minutes.

Serves 4.

★

RICH COCOA BROWNIES

PER BROWNIE: 168 CALORIES, 3.6 G PROTEIN, 21.4 G CARBOHYDRATE, 7.9 G FAT (3.9 G SATURATED),
22.6 MG SODIUM, 3.1 G FIBER, **PE CONTENT 0–5 MG**

8 tablespoons (4 ounces) unsalted butter
¼ cup honey
¼ cup pure maple syrup
1 teaspoon vanilla
⅓ cup unsweetened cocoa
1 cup chocolate-flavored soy milk
2½ cups whole-wheat pastry flour
¼ teaspoon baking powder
¼ cup chopped nuts (pecans, walnuts, almonds, or hazelnuts)

Preheat oven to 375° F.

Combine butter, honey, maple syrup, vanilla, and cocoa in small saucepan. Heat over medium heat until butter melts, whisking until smooth. Remove from heat and stir in soy milk.

Sift flour and baking powder into small bowl. Stir into cocoa mixture just until blended. Fold in nuts. Spoon batter into greased and floured 8-inch square baking pan. Bake at 375° F for 35 minutes, or until toothpick inserted in center of cake comes out clean.

Cool in pan on wire rack; cut into 2-inch squares.

Makes 16 brownies.

Recipe from *Healthy and Delicious Recipes, Vol. 1.* By permission of VitaSoy.

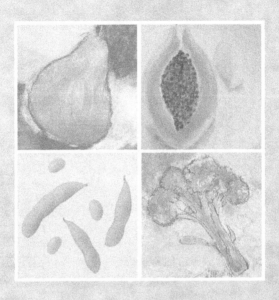

Appendix

Health Glossary

References

Resources

Index

Appendix

A simplified diagram showing the phytoestrogens that are currently known to be important to humans

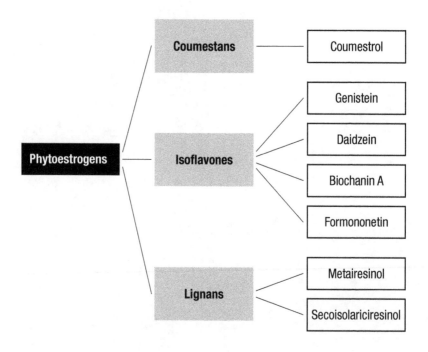

Note: Other, much less important phytoestrogens are omitted from the above diagram.

Health Glossary

(See page 79 for Glossary of Ingredients)

Alzheimer's disease A degenerative condition affecting the brain and leading to dementia.

antiangiogenic A substance that can prevent new blood vessels from forming, especially in a tumor. Rapidly growing tumors require a lot of nutrients for expansion and growth of their deviant cells, and nutrients are carried by the blood vessels. Thus, by stopping more blood vessels from growing around tumor sites, tumor growth is controlled.

antibacterial A substance that can fight against germs.

anticoagulant A substance that can thin or dissolve blood clots.

antiestrogenic A substance that can oppose the effects of estrogens.

antifungal A substance that can fight against fungus. A fungus belongs to the plant kingdom. An example of a fungus is candida.

antihypertensive A substance that can control or lower blood pressure.

anti-inflammatory A substance that can suppress or soothe inflamed parts of the body.

antioxidants Chemicals that can prevent oxidation of food products. These chemicals prevent free oxygen radicals from harming the body; for example, they can prevent formation of cholesterol plaques within blood vessels. Examples of common antioxidants are vitamins C and E.

antiviral A substance that can fight against viruses. An example of a virus is the common cold virus.

benign Mild in character. In medicine, a benign tumor is not malignant.

carcinogen Any substance that either promotes or initiates cancer.

carotenemia Excessive carotene in the body due to overconsumption of carotene-containing foods. Usually manifests itself by an orange-yellow skin; most evident on the palms of the hands.

cholesterol A fatlike substance produced by the liver or obtained from food. It is essential for the production of cell membranes, sex hormones, and vitamin D, among other things. High blood-cholesterol levels are often associated with an increased risk of heart disease.

coronary artery disease (CAD) A condition that may result in a heart attack. When the coronary arteries delivering blood to the heart become clogged with plaque, they can narrow and impair blood flow.

coumestans Chemicals that are structurally related to isoflavones and have estrogenic effects. These are found in plant products such as alfalfa, clover, soybean sprouts, and other legume sprouts.

daidzein Isoflavone found in soy that has been shown to have anticancer properties.

DVT Deep venous thrombosis. This refers to clots in the deep veins inside the legs.

equol A weak estrogen-like plant chemical, produced by bacterial action on phytoestrogens in the gut.

estradiol Female hormone found in the blood of premenopausal women.

estriol Female hormone found in the blood of pregnant women.

estrone Female hormone found in the blood of menopausal women.

fibroids Benign fleshy growths in the uterus (womb) that can cause problems with periods.

fluid retention Can cause feelings of puffiness in the legs and fingers, and is often accompanied by a bloated stomach. It can result from a number of causes. Women may notice this problem around the time when they expect their periods to arrive.

gastrointestinal Refers to the stomach, small bowel, and large bowel.

genistein A chemical found in soy that has very strong estrogenic effects as compared to the other plant estrogens. It has a strong anticancer effect on the body.

high-density lipoprotein (HDL) The body's major carrier of cholesterol to the liver for excretion in bile. Often referred to as "good cholesterol."

hormone replacement therapy (HRT) Treating a hormone-deficiency state with prescription hormones. In the context of this book, it refers to estrogens, given either alone or in combination with a progesterone.

isoflavones Compounds found in some plant products, which have estrogenic properties. These products' structure differs slightly from that of coumestans. Genistein and daidzein are examples of isoflavones.

legumes This food group includes fresh and dried beans, peas, lentils, and kidney beans.

low-density lipoprotein (LDL) Believed to take cholesterol from the blood and deposit it in the cells. Called "bad cholesterol" because studies indicate that high levels of LDL enhance the risk of developing CAD (see top of previous page).

menopause Refers to a woman's last natural menstrual period. For most women, it is a retrospective label. A woman is said to have gone through menopause if she hasn't had a period in the preceding twelve months. If she still has a period every three to four months, or even every six months, she has not yet reached menopause.

menses Monthly menstrual periods.

metabolism Burning of energy to maintain cell function.

nausea A feeling of sickness in the stomach or belly, accompanied by an urge to throw up the stomach's contents.

osteoporosis Thinning of bone with loss of bone mineral density. It can result in easy fractures with or without minimal trauma.

Pap smear Sampling of cells from the cervix (mouth of the womb) to detect early cervical cancer.

perimenopause Years immediately preceding menopause (see above). Perimenopausal women may experience irregularity in their periods, accompanied by some menopausal symptoms such as hot flashes, mood changes, and sleeplessness.

phytic acid A chemical present in some plant products that can bind up minerals such as zinc, calcium, iron, etc. If it is ingested in large quantities, a person may experience cramps at night.

phytoestrogens Naturally occurring compounds with estrogenic properties found in some plants. Phytoestrogens are similar in structure to human
estrogens, but their effects are very weak compared to those of human
estrogens.

premenopause Years of a woman's life before menopause.

progesterone The other female hormone produced by the ovaries.
In general, progesterone has antiestrogenic effects.

protease inhibitor A chemical that blocks the action of specific enzymes
thought to be responsible in the formation or growth of tumors.

tempeh A fermented soybean product that has a meaty, nutty taste. It is
rich in proteins, iron, calcium, and B-group vitamins.

tofu Soybean curd made from concentrated soy milk, with a coagulant
added to set the mixture. Weight for weight, tofu is less concentrated in
nutrients than tempeh.

transit time Time taken for the passage of a food item. In the context
of this book, refers to the time the item takes to pass through the digestive
system.

triglycerides A type of fat that is manufactured by the liver and obtained
from dietary fat. Triglycerides circulate in the bloodstream and are either
used for energy or stored in body tissues as fat. Elevated levels are common
in coronary artery disease.

References

Adami, S., et al. 1997. Ipriflavone prevents radial bone loss in postmenopausal women with low bone mass over two years. *Osteoporosis International* 7(2):119–25.

Adlercreutz, H. 1995. Phytoestrogens: Epidemiology and a possible role in cancer protection. *Environmental Health Perspectives* 103 (Supplement 7):103–12.

Adlercreutz, H. 1996. Phytoestrogens from biochemistry to prevention of cancer and other diseases. Eighth International Congress on the Menopause Symposium, Sydney, Australia.

Adlercreutz, H., et al. 1992. Dietary phyto-oestrogens and menopause in Japan. *The Lancet* 339:1233.

Agnusdei, D., et al. 1992. Effects of ipriflavone on bone mass and calcium metabolism in postmenopausal osteoporosis. *Bone and Mineral* 19 (Supplement 1):S43–48.

Albert, A., et al. 2002. Efficacy and safety of a phytoestrogen preparation derived from glycine max (L.) merr in climacteric symptomatology: A multicentric, open, prospective and non-randomized trial. *Phytomedicine* 9(2):85–92.

Albertazzi, Paola, et al. 1998. The effect of dietary soy supplementation on hot flushes. *Obstetrics and Gynecology* 91(1):6–11.

Alexandersen, P., et al. 2001. Ipriflavone in the treatment of postmenopausal osteoporosis: A randomized controlled trial. *Journal of the American Medical Association* 285(11):142–48.

Anderson, J. J. B., and S. C. Garner. 1997. The effects of phytoestrogens on bone. *Nutrition Research* 17:1617–32.

Anderson, J. W., et al. 1995. Meta-analysis of the effects of soy protein intake on serum lipids. *New England Journal of Medicine* 333:276–82.

Baird, D. D., et al. 1995. Dietary intervention study to assess estrogenicity of dietary soy among postmenopausal women. *Journal of Clinical Endocrinology and Metabolism* 8:1685–90.

Bierenbaum, Marvin, et al. 1994. Reducing atherogenic risk in hyperlipemic humans with flaxseed supplementation: A preliminary report. *American College of Nutrition* 12(5):501–4.

Black, C. 1994. Menopause: The alternative way. *Australian Women's Research Centre* 1:62–80.

Boulet, M. J. 1994. Climacteric and menopause in seven south-east Asian countries. *Maturitas* 19:157–76.

Bungay, T., et al. 1980. Study of symptoms in middle life with special reference to the menopause. *British Medical Journal* 281:181–83.

Caroll, K. K. 1991. Review of clinical studies on cholesterol-lowering response to soy protein. *Journal of the American Dietary Association* 91:820.

Carper, J. 1993. *Food: Your Miracle Medicine.* New York: HarperCollins Publishers.

Cashel, K., R. English, and J. Lewis. 1989. *Composition of Foods.* Australia: Australian Government Publishing Service.

Cassidy, A., et al. 1994. Biological effects of a diet of soy protein rich in isofla-vones on the menstrual cycle of premenopausal women. *American Journal of Clinical Nutrition* 60:333–40.

Colditz, Graham, et al. 1995. The use of estrogens and progestins and the risk of breast cancer in postmenopausal women. *New England Journal of Medicine* 332:1589–93.

Cunnane, Stephen C., et al. 1993. High alpha-linolenic acid flaxseed (*Linum usi-tatissimum*): Some nutritional properties in humans. *British Journal of Nutrition* 69:443–53.

———. 11 April 1995. Current concepts in the early detection of breast cancer. Third Annual Oncology Conference: American Cancer Society.

———. 1995. Nutritional attributes of traditional flaxseed in healthy young adults. *American Journal of Clinical Nutrition* 61:62–68.

Dalais, F. S., et al. 1996. The effects of phytoestrogens in postmenopausal women. Eighth International Congress on the Menopause Symposium, Sydney, Australia.

Dennerstein, L., et al. 1993. Menopausal symptoms in Australian women. *Medical Journal of Australia* 159:232–36.

Draper, C. R., et al. 1997. Phytoestrogens reduce bone loss and bone resorption in oophorectomized rats. *Journal of Nutrition* 127(9):1795–99.

Dwyer, Johanna, et al. 1994. Tofu and soy drinks contain phytoestrogens. *Journal of the American Dietary Association* 94:739–43.

Eden, J. A. 1992. Oestrogen and the breast: The management of the menopausal woman with breast cancer. *Medical Journal of Australia* 157:247–49.

Eden, J. A., et al. 1996. A controlled trial of isoflavones for menopausal symp-toms. Eighth International Congress on the Menopause Symposium, Sydney, Australia.

Edington, R. F., et al. 1980. Clonidine (Dixarit) for menopausal flushing. *Canadian Medical Association Journal* 123:23–26.

Erdman, J. W., and S. M. Potter. 1997. Soy and bone health. *Soy Connect* 5:1.

Fraser, Gary E. 1994. Diet and coronary heart disease: Beyond dietary fats and low-density-lipoprotein cholesterol. *American Journal of Clinical Nutrition* 59 (Suppl.):1117S–23S.

Gaddi, Antonio, et al. 1991. Dietary treatment for familian hypercholesterolemia: Differential effects of dietary soy protein according to the apolipoprotein E phenotypes. *American Journal of Clinical Nutrition* 53:1191–96.

Gambacciani, M., et al. 1993. Effects of ipriflavone administration on bone mass and metabolism in ovariectomized women. *Journal of Endocrinological Investigation* 16(5):333–37.

Gennari, C., et al. 1997. Effect of chronic treatment with ipriflavone in post-menopausal women with low bone mass. *Calcified Tissue International* 61 (Supplement 1):S19–22.

Goldin, B. R. 1994. Nonsteroidal estrogens and estrogen antagonists: Mechanisms of action and health implications. *Journal of the National Cancer Institute* 86:174.

Goodman, Marc, et al. 1997. Association of soy and fiber consumption with the risk of endometrial cancer. *American Journal of Epidemiology* 146:294–306.

Greenstein, J., et al. 1996. Risk of breast cancer associated with intake of specific foods and food groups. *American Journal of Epidemiology* 143(11):S36.

Griffiths, K. 1996. Epidemiology of phytoestrogens, cancer and other diseases. Eighth International Congress on the Menopause Symposium, Sydney, Australia.

Hasler, Clare, and Susan Calvert Finn. 1998. Soy: Just a hill of beans? *Journal of Women's Health* 7(5):519–23.

Herman, C., et al. 1995. Soybean phytoestrogen intake and cancer risk. *Journal of Nutrition* 125:757S–70S.

Hernandez-Avita, M., et al. 1991. Caffeine, moderate alcohol intake, and risk of fractures of the hip and forearm in middle-aged women. *American Journal of Clinical Nutrition* 54(1):157–63.

Hoidrup, S., et al. 1999. Alcohol intake, beverage preference, and risk of hip fracture in men and women. Copenhagen Center for Prospective Studies. *American Journal of Epidemiology* 149(1):939–1001.

Hughes, C. J. 1996. Phytoestrogens. Eighth International Congress on the Menopause Symposium, Sydney, Australia.

Hully, Stephen, et al. 1998. Randomized trial of estrogen plus progestin for secondary prevention of coronary heart disease in postmenopausal women. *Journal of the American Medical Association* 280(7):605–13.

Hutchins, Andrea, et al. 1995. Vegetables, fruits, and legumes: Effect on urinary isoflavonoid phytoestrogen and lignan excretion. *Journal of the American Dietary Association* 95:769–74.

Ingram, David, et al. 1994. Just the flax, ma'am: Researchers testing linseed. *Journal of the National Cancer Institute* 86:1746–47.

———. 1997. Case-control study of phyto-oestrogens and breast cancer. *The Lancet* 350:990–94.

Knight, D. C., and J. Eden. 1995. Phytoestrogens: A short review. *Maturitus* 22:167–75.

Knight, D. C., et al. 1996. A review of the clinical effects of phytoestrogens. *Obstetrics and Gynecology* 87:897–904.

Lampe, Johanna, et al. 1994. Urinary lignan and isoflavonoid excretion in premenopausal women consuming flaxseed powder. *American Journal of Clinical Nutrition* 60:122–28.

Lacey, J., et al. 2002. Menopausal hormone replacement therapy and risk of ovarian cancer. *Journal of the American Medical Association.* 288(3):334–41.

Lee, H. P., et al. 1991. Dietary effects on breast-cancer risks in Singapore. *The Lancet* 337:1197–200.

Little, B. 1986. *The Complete Book of Herbs and Spices.* New South Wales, Australia: Reed Books.

Llewellyn-Jones, D., and S. Abrahams. 1988. *Menopause.* Victoria, Australia: Ashwood House/Penguin Books, 65–75.

Louria, D. B., et al. 1985. Onion extract in treatment of hypertension and hyperlipidemia: A preliminary communication. *Current Therapeutic Research* 37:127–31.

Mazur, W. 1998. Phytoestrogen content in foods. *Balliere's Clinical Endocrinology and Metabolism* 12(4):729–42.

Messina, Mark, and Stephen Barnes. 1991. The role of soy products in reducing risk of cancer. *Journal of the National Cancer Institute* 83(8):541–46.

Messina, Mark, et al. 1997. Phyto-oestrogens and breast cancer. *The Lancet* 350:971–72.

Murkies, A. L., et al. 1995. Dietary flour supplementation decreases postmenopausal hot flushes: Effect of soy and wheat. *Maturitus* 21:189–95.

National Health and Medical Research Council. 1992. *Dietary Guidelines for Australians.* Australia: Australian Government Publishing Service.

Potter, S. M. 1995. Overview of proposed mechanisms for the hypocholesterolemic effect of soy. *Journal of Nutrition* 125:606S.

Prince, R. 1993. The calcium controversy revisited: Implications of new data. *Medical Journal of Australia* 159:404–6.

Riggs, B. L., and I. J. Melton. 1992. The prevention and treatment of osteoporosis. *New England Journal of Medicine* 327(9):602–27.

Rossouw, J. E., et al. 2002. Risks and benefits of estrogen plus progestin in healthy postmenopausal women. *Journal of the American Medical Association.* 288(3):321–33.

Sack, M. N., et al. 1994. Oestrogen and inhibition of oxidation of low-density lipoproteins in postmenopausal women. *Lancet* 343:269–70.

Saltman, D. 1994. *In Transition: A Guide to Menopause.* New South Wales, Australia: Choice Books.

Shumaker, S. A., et al. 2003. Estrogen plus progestin and the incidence of dementia and mild cognitive impairment in postmenopausal women. *Journal of the American Medical Association* 289(20):2651–62.

Sojka, J. E., and C. M. Weaver. 1995. Magnesium supplementation and osteoporosis. *Nutrition Reviews* 53(3):71–74.

Somekawa, Y., et al. 2001. Soy intake related to menopausal symptoms, serum lipids, and bone mineral density in postmenopausal Japanese women. *Obstetrics and Gynecology* 97(1):109–15.

Stanton, R. 1989. *The Complete Book of Food and Nutrition*. Sydney, Australia: Simon and Schuster.

Stuart, M. 1982. *The Color Dictionary of Herbs and Herbalism*. London: Orbis Publishing.

Upmalis, D. H., et al. 2000. Vasomotor symptom relief by soy isoflavone extract tablets in postmenopausal women: A multicenter, double-blind, randomized, placebo-controlled study. *Menopause* 7(4):236–42.

Van Schaick, S. 1993. Symptomatic treatment of hot flushes. *Therapeutics Update* 61–65.

Vines, G. 1994. Cancer: Is soy the solution? *New Scientist* July:14–15.

Wilcox, G. 1996. Effect of soy on menopausal symptoms. Eighth International Congress on the Menopause Symposium, Sydney, Australia.

Wilcox, G., et al. 1990. Oestrogenic effects of plant foods in postmenopausal women. *British Medical Journal* 30:905–6.

Wolk, Alicja, et al. 1998. A prospective study of association of monounsaturated fat and other types of fat with risk of breast cancer. *Archives of Internal Medicines* 158:41–45.

Zandi P. P., et al. 2002. Hormone replacement therapy and the incidence of Alzheimer disease in older women: the Cache County Study. *Journal of the American Medical Association* 288 (17):2123–29.

Resources

⤛ Information on Soy Products ⤜

The U.S. Soyfoods Directory

Sponsored by the Indiana Soybean Board
  E-mail: info@soyfoods.com
  Website: www.soyfoods.com

⤛ Specialty Soy Products ⤜

Revival Soy Products

Revival sells soy shakes, soy protein bars, soy nuts, soy pasta, and other soy foods, all specially formulated to contain high amounts of phytoestrogens. Revival products are unavailable in stores; they must be ordered directly from the company.

  Customer Service: (800) 500-1297
  Ordering: (800) REVIVAL (738-4825)
  Website: www.revivalsoy.com

⤛ Natural Progesterone Creams ⤜

Pro-Gest

(800) 888-6814
  Website: www.emerita.com (Emerita is the retail division of Transitions for Health, manufacturers of Pro-Gest)

FemGest

  Website: www.femgest.com

⤳ Mail-Order Sources for Recipe Ingredients ⤳

Penzeys Spices

Complete line of dried spices including Chinese five-spice blend, Indian garam masala blend, dried lemongrass, star anise, curry powders.

(800) 741-7787
Website: www.penzeys.com

Richters Herb Specialists

Major source of herb seeds and live plants, including dried herbs of many types. Source for licorice root (dried roots, seeds), dong quai (live plants or seeds), and lemongrass (live plants or powdered).

(905) 640-6677
Website: www.richters.com

Uwajimaya

Asian food and gift market. Featuring Japanese, Chinese, and Korean food products and equipment.

(206) 624-6248
Website: www.uwajimaya.com

Index

Boldface page numbers refer to recipes located in the text.